DEPRESSION WEARS LIPSTICK

1

for the depressed, broken, abused and silenced.
You are not alone.

I dedicate this book to:

Della Browning (MamaB)
Yolanda Morrow
Suddie Scott
Trish Nickolas
Lori D. Taylor

Depression Wears Lipstick
Toi Nichelle
Copyright © 2019
Dream Loud Ink, Publishing

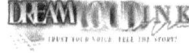

ISBN: 0-9786817-1-1
        978-0-9786817-1-5

Published by (DLI) Dream Loud Ink, Publishing
Toi Nichelle
Typeset & Editing by: Dream Loud Ink, Publishing
Email : Dreamloudinc@yahoo.com

Other Works by Toi Nichelle:

◆━━━━━━━━◆

Mirror to my Soul ~ A Poetry Anthology © 2007
The Hush Language ~ A Poet's Memoir © 2010
The Scholarship Thief ~ Undergrad Edition © 2016

PRAISE FOR DEPRESSION WEARS LIPSTICK

"*Depression Wears Lipstick* is an intriguing inquiry on how one woman fought depression and suicide by revisiting her past to explore a better future. *Depression Wears Lipstick* connects with an audience from all walks of life, while showing you how to overcome."

Dream Loud Ink, Publishing

"I am floored. This is an excellent book, very well written. Not only does it outline your challenges and trials, but it also gives solutions to the problems, a road map to restoration, forgiveness, success, love and loving yourself. I am feeling so blessed to know you."

Tammy Doss, Executive Officer
Dream Loud Ink, Publishing

"It is amazing to see just how much God has worked with you. You have become a very inspirational young lady for all to follow. Not only has God helped heal you, but he has made it so now you are inspiring and lifting up others. You are a true testimony and blessing to us all. I am so proud to call you my dear friend."

Yolanda Morrow
Los Angeles, California

"I had the absolute pleasure to experience an excerpt from *Depression Wears Lipstick: Depression Will Kill You, written by Toi Nichelle.* This book is a no non-sense read. One learns what depression is and it is alive and well and often where you least expect to find it; in the church – the Lord's house. Toi shares her experience of this disorder. She makes it clear to the reader it is a feeling(s) that can take over if not treated. But there is hope. Read this honest, heart-warming beautiful account of a persistent feeling of sadness and loss of interest…but God!

Yvetta D. Franklin
Author & Tenured Educator

TABLE OF CONTENTS

THE PAST

CHAPTERS 1-4

THE PRESENT

CHAPTERS 5-8

THE FUTURE

CHAPTERS 9-18

INFORMATION

Dealing with Depression? Dealing with Suicide?

SUICIDE HOTLINE:

(800) 273-8255

Further resource list at end of book

Disclaimer

This book is meant to be a useful aid of encouragement and motivation during the difficult times of depression. No form of this book is to be copied and pasted. Plagiarism is against the law.

I am in no way proclaiming to be an expert, therefore, the information you see in this book is based on life experiences of the author. Although experiences are different based on an individual's circumstance, the information given in this book may be helpful to someone. If you are experiencing symptoms of depression, stress or suicide, please seek profession help. Remember, your life is important, and no one will know you need help unless you speak up.

Please, as you read this book, use what is helpful and research on your own for other information you may need on how to deal and cope with depression.

Five Stages of Depression

This pyramid is my perception of depression and how I noticed it in myself. These stages have not been scientifically proven, but have appeared to be a constant theme in people I have known to battle with depression. I am using this as an example of how severe it can become for an individual.

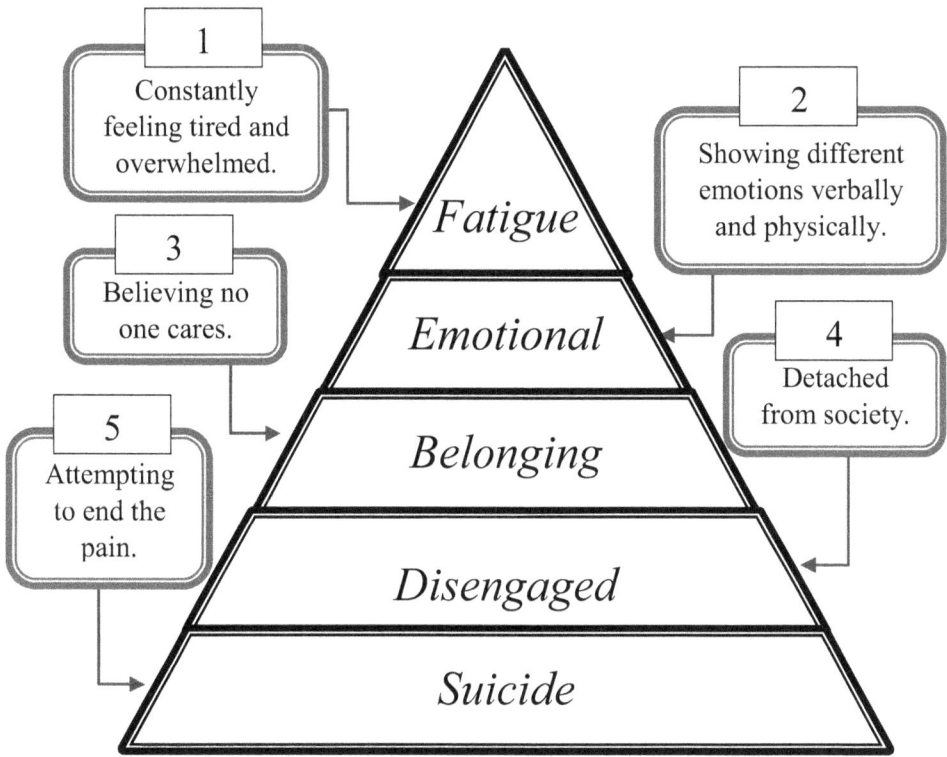

1 Constantly feeling tired and overwhelmed.

2 Showing different emotions verbally and physically.

3 Believing no one cares.

4 Detached from society.

5 Attempting to end the pain.

Fatigue

Emotional

Belonging

Disengaged

Suicide

On the next page, I describe how these stages were constant in my life, and how they kept me from living my full potential. As you read them and see signs within yourself, please take some time to work through them, and get professional help if necessary.

Fatigue

Problem

At one point in my life I noticed that I was constantly tired. I would get a full eight hours of sleep, but still felt overwhelmed. I remember going to the doctor and finding out that I had fibroid tumors in my uterus, which caused me to have heavy cycles during that time of the month. I know this may seem like 'too much information' but it's necessary. After going to the doctor and discovering this ailment, I was then informed that I had low anemia due to the blood loss and insufficient iron, and may need a blood transfusion.

Cause

Clearly, this was the cause of my tiredness and I overlooked the deeper problem I was experiencing. I realized that not only was I fatigued from low iron, but I was actively living with depression and it drained my energy.

Action

When I discovered this, I began to focus on my medical and mental needs, often exploring rest as a healing device. Find out what is causing you to be more tired than usual. It may just be a health situation, but sometimes, there is an underlying theme to your health that goes beyond what is visible.

Emotional

Problem

I have always been a sensitive person. I was taught to be closed in and "secretive" as my mother calls me. I realized that I was this way because my upbringing didn't allow me to explore conversation and express what I dealt with as a child. We didn't talk to each other and because of this, the Great Wall of China was built between us. In school, I was bullied and tormented until I cried, or hid in a corner alone.

| Cause |

This caused me to be more emotional than 'normal', and I didn't understand how to direct this energy. One day I was happy, singing joyful songs unto the Lord; the next day, I was crying with pills in my hand, contemplating on ending it all.

| Action |

I went to therapy. This is when I realized that happiness shouldn't be a temporary emotion, but there are many of us who are experiencing it. Try keeping track of when you feel your emotions are jumping from one feeling to the next. You'll most likely see a pattern that causes you to get emotional when you should be happy.

Belonging

| Problem |

Being homeless at an early age and living from pillar to post, caused me to feel misplaced. I felt like no one wanted me, and no matter how hard I tried, I was put out because of my quietness and not knowing how to communicate properly. My mom overworked herself until she gave up; my father abandoned his responsibilities and then passed away, and my sisters never accepted me and were partly the reasons I wanted to die.

| Cause |

As an adult, I continued feeling like no one cared for me and I didn't belong anywhere. I felt helpless and thought that I didn't have purpose for my life.

| Action |

Purpose came in undergrad. I was at San Francisco State University and realized that I had a divine opportunity to live without limits. I took baby steps and discovered that with each step, I am a walking miracle. If you are feeling like you don't belong anywhere, maybe it's because you are not supposed to fit into a box. You can't breathe in a box, so get out of it. Take baby steps, and find your inner strength.

Disengaged

Problem

I felt alone because most times I made myself feel alone. Depression will make you feel like there is no one you can talk to when you need it the most. I would constantly pull away from people because that's all I knew how to do. If they didn't show up like they said, or failed to keep their promise, I would pull back and become 'detached' emotionally. I was used to everyone in my family hurting and pushing me away, so I was no stranger to this.

Cause

It became my 'safety mechanism', if you will. If I felt like I was being hurt, I would run for the hills, never looking back. I would often say that I am a 'homebody' because I didn't like any attention to come my way. I didn't want to go out and be around people. I am somewhat of an introvert. I can only handle large amounts of people for a certain period of time before I need to be alone and recharge.

Action

I started going out more. I made plans with the people I was close to and we started going out to dinner or coffee. This gave me a sense of engagement and helped with my social anxiety. If you are constantly finding yourself wanting to stay in bed, get up and call a friend. Make plans to go out, even if it's just to window shop.

Suicide

Problem
I don't like this word, but we overlook it until that person who showed deep signs of depression is found dead. I will not lie just because I am supposed to be the strong one. There were numerous times I wanted to die, and even attempted it. My upbringing played a major role in this for me, and I hit a crossroad where I had to make a choice.

Cause
Suicide scared me because the last thing I wanted to do was create this legacy of death in my life. I wrote death threats to myself, and asked God to kill me in my prayers. This was my cry for help! I am so glad I serve a God who knows our heart issues, and doesn't always give us what we ask for.

Action
I had to apologize to God, first, then to myself. It can get tough for most of us, but isn't it worth seeing this thing called life to the end? We all will die someday. Why expedite your grave and invest in your headstone before it's time? The biggest help you can give yourself is to seek professional help. Call the suicide hotline and speak to someone. I am glad I made the choice to voice my struggle, instead of killing all that I am becoming.

QUESTIONNAIRE

This questionnaire is designed to put you in the right mind in understanding where you are in your journey. If it does not apply, simply check *NO,* but if you feel that you can relate, check *YES.*

1. Are there signs you see within yourself that causes you to be depressed?

    ☐YES   ☐NO

2. Are you holding onto things from your past?

    ☐YES   ☐NO

3. Are there any family secrets you are tired of keeping?

    ☐YES   ☐NO

4. Have you ever been sexually abused?

    ☐YES   ☐NO

5. Have you considered professional help?

    ☐YES   ☐NO

6. Are you suicidal? Or have you ever considered suicide?

    ☐YES   ☐NO

7. Are you tired of living in the past?

    ☐YES   ☐NO

8. Are you ready to take some steps to overcome?

    ☐YES   ☐NO

9. Are you searching for purpose in your life?

    ☐YES   ☐NO

PRAYER FOR OVERCOMING DEPRESSION

Dear Heavenly Father,

We first come to you acknowledging that you are God, and that there is no one who sits higher than you.

We come asking for forgiveness of our daily sins that we commit, knowingly and unknowingly.

We understand and believe in our hearts that if we confess with our mouths you are able and righteous to forgive and pardon us from the heavy loads we carry.

We believe that you are the same God who delivers and heals, so we ask of your healing power to reign in our lives.

We petition heaven to help us overcome the vile attacks of the enemy on our lives.

We pray that you open a clearing in our minds to be transformed into all things good and perfect.

We understand that everyone's journey is different, but we believe that there is only one supernatural power of God that can sustain us.

We pray for every reader, that as they begin to interpret the chapters and turn the pages, shackles are being loosed off their lives and the chains are broken.

We believe that depression has no authority to occupy our minds, therefore we cast it back to whence it came.

We stand in agreement that your supernatural healing will begin to manifest in the readers lives and they'll believe in the victory that is already theirs for the taking.

Amen.

"Depressed people live in the past.

People with anxiety live in the future.

Happy people live in the present."

– Unknown

I come to find that if I section my life in these three parts I can begin the true healing process and discover what is keeping me stagnant today.

So, let's start off with the past. What happened in my past that has gotten me so depressed even now as an adult?

The Past

DEPRESSED PEOPLE LIVE IN THE PAST

"There are two great days in a person's life - the day we are born and the day we discover why." William Barclay

1

WHEN DEPRESSION BECAME REAL

"I believe the struggle of what you're mentally dealing with can make you sick, drain you and keep you waiting on a memory which no longer exists; and can ultimately lead to your demise."

*I*t is sometimes feminine and educated. It does not appear to be in shambles, but it is a teacher of life. It finds joy in wanting to help others, but desperately needs the reciprocation. It does not always appear to be what you think it should be. It can sometimes come from a good family or not so good family. It masks itself in becoming real in what you need in the moment. It is an illusion. It is your truth.

I never thought that I would be able to admit that I have suffered from depression for years. I titled this book, *Depression Wears Lipstick,* because sometimes it's hard to tell just by looking at a person if they are dealing with depression. Like myself, depression was feminine and educated, who sometimes wore pink lipstick. I am not ashamed of my journey because I recognize who I am becoming. I have noticed that most people do not want to hear the truth. They want to know that you are "yet holding on", but don't want to hear the deep struggles you may be facing. Depression is not something to play with, so you must be careful who you share your journey with. You also must understand that most people will not get your condition, which causes them to mishandle, but they really don't understand the depth of it.

When I first realized that depression was real, I was an undergrad at San Francisco State University and working at my 9-5 job, so I just equated it to working and going to school. I figured that I was just a little bit stressed out and *"this too shall pass"* as we say in the church. After a while, once I graduated with my degree and got a job it did not pass. It became more real in my life than anyone else around me. I don't know about you but my depression spoke to me. My depression looked at me in the mirror and called my name with a familiar voice that I had no choice but to answer it. I'm not telling you all of this just for the sake of it, but I'm saying this because sometimes we think people who are depressed look depressed and that is not often the case. I was always encouraging people to go after their dreams and goals in life. I wanted to see people happy but often wondered if people's real intent was to see me happy as well. I know you may be thinking, *"girl you have to love yourself and don't worry about what other people have to say"*. Those are two clichés that we tend to say, and oftentimes it's more than not loving yourself or not caring about what other people have to say, but it deals more with figuring out the balance in your life and understanding that sometimes loving yourself will not always be a good day. Sometimes you love yourself to the core but everything around you is going wrong and it makes you a little sad. It doesn't mean that you do not love yourself; it just means that it is difficult right now. It means there are some battles you must face so that you can get over them.

I understand that there may be some people out there who equate not loving yourself with being depressed. I agree to an extent because there are a variety of people who experience depression and hate who they are. I cannot say that I hated myself to the core, but I hated what I went through and what I allowed myself to go through. So yes, there are people who hate themselves and are depressed, and there are those who love themselves but struggle with depression because they have not dealt with the issue. This can considerably be argued, but we're not here for arguments. I am writing this because I know what it feels like to struggle with depression, and this internal battle to survive.

My goal in this book is to break down how I dealt with depression. The things I am about to reveal does not come from a professional. I am not claiming to be a therapist, and it may not seem politically correct to some, but it is my truth. This book is not meant to be a tell all. I am in no way harboring the past while looking for attention. I will say that as a person who has dealt with depression, it is easy to be put in a box. Let me reveal something to you: *we can't breathe in a box, and dealing with depression is hard enough.* As you read this book, become more sensitive to those around you, and understand that we are fighting.

WHEN DID DEPRESSION BECOME REAL FOR YOU?

_____

_____

_____

_____

_____

_____

_____

_____

_____

2

DEPRESSION WILL KILL YOU!

"I do not want my thoughts to die with me;
therefore, I ask that you listen."

Depression will destroy what little happiness you have, if you let it. I had to learn the hard way, and it was not easy admitting it because most times when I admitted my struggles in the church, I often got a response like this, "Just pray about it." I agree with this response. Pray about it. But what happens when you pray about it, and it becomes heavier to deal with? Most people in the church are not equipped to deal with depression. I agree with this as well. One thing I can say is that when you are actively experiencing depression, you do not quite comprehend this type of response, and wish that people would be more understanding. It isn't until your eyes are opened that you realize, you must fight this internal battle alone, without people, and sometimes the much-needed spiritual guidance.

> *"It is easy to believe lies when you*
> *have never been told the truth."*

Most of my depression started in my childhood, where insecurities of feeling unloved and unwanted by family was heavy. As I got older, the word *family* did not mean anything to me because I have never felt what family was capable of being. I only experienced the damage that family could do. How it destroys your thought pattern, and makes you believe that you are worthless. *It is a trick of the enemy!* Being older, I realize that most things I went through as a child; sexual abuse, mental abuse, verbal abuse and suicidal attempts, I never really dealt with it like I thought I had. I brushed over it and tried to do things to sort of make my life feel better for the moment because the truth is, I didn't feel better. I didn't feel good about my life. I didn't feel good about who I was. I felt that I was ugly because the verbal abuse I experienced growing up told me so. When I looked in the mirror, I saw a monster. I saw someone who couldn't be loved, someone who had all these flaws that was pointed out to me daily by family and friends, and somewhere down the line I started to believe those lies. It is easy to believe lies when you have never been told the truth. I didn't find out the truth until later in life. When I finally discovered the truth about myself, I struggled even harder. Here I was learning that I was beautiful in the sight of God, learning to see beauty in myself, and I struggled being a woman of faith not knowing how to overcome the previous lies. For years, I felt like an outcast in the church growing up. Church was supposed to be a place that you could go when you're hurting and in pain, but oftentimes when you get to church, you're afraid to show those scars because the judgement is right there at the front door. This does not happen at every church, but in my opinion, it shouldn't happen at any church.

It was difficult admitting it because what I have experienced in the church is that you get stoned, not in a literal sense, for saying what you're dealing with. I am not saying every church or Christian faith is like this or that it happens all the time, but I have experienced it. For example, there have been times that I have sought out spiritual counseling regarding my depression and wanting to die. I have been told, "Jesus died for your sins and God can make it all better. He'll be your comforter in the darkest times." I believe every single one of those words because I have truly felt the comfort and protection of God during those times when I felt like I was not going to make it. I believe those words to my core. I also believe that when you have been traumatized as a child, someone sexually hurting you and telling you that if you told they'll do something to you, at some point you must deal with that mental issue. I had to learn that I carried this cross for far too long. Dear reader: *You have carried the cross of silence long enough.*

It was not until a few years ago, I realized my mental health was off balance. I was doing more damage to myself because I could not talk about it, which was frustrating to me. I chose to speak up about certain things I was dealing with regardless if people or the church liked it, or not. I didn't want to live a lie, but I also didn't want to feel like I was conjuring up the past. With this realization, my true journey began. Peace was waiting for me, but in order to get it, I had to start from the beginning. I had to fight when I felt like there was no fight left in me.

This might sound difficult to hear for some, but I remember having a conversation with a friend about depression in the church. I revealed to her that on more than a few occasions the pastor would do an altar call. He would say, "if you've ever felt like giving up, or committing suicide, come to the altar." On plenty occasions, I would go up to the altar followed by a crowd of individuals who wanted to kill themselves. When we arrived at the altar, the pastor would pray, maybe lay his hands on us, and at the end send us on our merry way. Everyone that came to the altar had to go home and face their suicidal thoughts, alone.

I remember one day I went to the altar in hopes of getting help. This particular morning, I had made it up in my mind that I wanted to die, but I would go to church first, then attempt afterwards. I experienced the same altar call, quick prayer, and a touch of oil on my forehead. After service, I felt worse than the moment I entered the church that morning. I ran to my car, cried my eyes out, started my car and debated on how I was going to drive my car into a river, off a cliff, head-on into a tree at full speed. I sat in my car with the engine running for a while wanting to be free from this feeling.

If you do not understand depression you might say, "don't wait on the church to help you, learn to help yourself." Good observation. What I can say is that depression, depending on what level you're on, works against those thoughts. I would also debate the existence of the church.

If the congregation is filled with suicidal members scattered throughout the pews, what is the church going to do about it? Should there be church partnerships with the community and various organizations dealing with mental health to help combat these attacks? Or should you just pretend to be happy and go to church, sit in the pew, sing in the choir and join various ministries until one day depression gets the best of you and your suicidal attempts are now actualized? There were times when I was scared for my life because no matter how hard I tried, coming to church Sunday after Sunday, I was struggling inside. It did not matter who I talked to in the church, I was always sent off with a scripture and quick prayer. There was never any follow-up calls or mental health service referrals given to me. I struggled very deeply because I knew inside I did not want to die, but was afraid of what I was capable of.

I believe this need to change in our church's, but like always the church will say, "you need to pray harder and build a relationship with God." Do you not know that when a person is dealing with depression, schizophrenia, suicide, bipolar and any other form of psychosis, not only do they need prayer, they need help? I have never been bipolar or schizophrenic, but I have experienced heavy depression and suicidal thoughts. It is all in the mental health category, and even the lowest level of depression deserves attention. If you are around someone who may be experiencing depression and questioning their life, please I beg of you, pay attention to the signs, the small hints they are dropping.

I remember dropping hints by texting certain people that I needed to talk. If I called them, they would forward me to voicemail. Sometimes, I would not get a response until days later, which would send me into a deeper depression. When I finally got a text response back it would sound something like this, *"hey girl, sorry I'm just now getting back to you. I've been busy."* A response like this can drive a depressed suicidal person over the edge. I have gotten stronger over the years, but must say that if we keep using this "I'm busy" response when someone is saying they need to speak to you, you might as well go purchase their headstone and dig up their burial plot. I know what it means to be busy, but life should not be so consuming that we fail to see those hints in a text message. If someone says they need to speak to me, I will try my best to make it urgent that I return their call, if I am capable. You never know what a person is going through, this is why I have learned some techniques on how to help myself. If I never get a response from my text message, I am no longer mentally running to jump off a cliff. If you want to be real about it, not getting a response will be someone's trigger to pick up that bottle of pills, go into the room, and die. Reaching out to that person lets them see that someone acknowledges and sees what they are going through, and most importantly, they are ready to listen.

What I have learned is that you can help ease a depressed suicidal person off the edge by acts of kindness, conversation and helping them to create a safe place to admit their struggles. If you are someone they hold close or in high regard, trust me when I say, listening and allowing them to be open with what they're dealing with matters.

ARE YOU EXPERIENCING DEPRESSION? HOW ARE YOU HANDLING IT?

3

LOW-TOLERANCE FOR TOUCHING

"I have learned that being ashamed brings greater pain than the actual past and the best thing you can do to overcome is to openly overcome."

I hate to admit it, though I have talked about it before in my previous book, *The Hush Language.* I titled it that because my adolescent years were filled with quiet lips, rambling thoughts, the first touch that turned into so much more and the games that were not so innocent. This is my beginning. Times when mom worked two jobs, and dad was like so many dads, invisible. With not much supervision, sexual spirits were invited into the home. I don't know how they got there. Not sure just how deep it goes, but I will say that my mother finally admitted something to me. She said in a letter labeled: PLEASE READ, "I was violated by an older man when I was younger." This is just an excerpt from the letter, but it made me realize that this sexual abuse made its way from the generation before me, and no one stopped it. No one protected my mother, so she may not have known how to protect her children. I can only imagine. I also realized that if my mother was violated, did my grandmother have a similar story? Where did it originate? These are questions I cannot fully answer, but I can stop it with me. The abuse started with family, and continued to happen to me by a male family *friend.*

As a three-year-old, experiencing someone touch you, you do not quite understand what is happening, but the way the conscious works, it tells you that something is not right. There were a whole lot of people that touched each other in my family. The incest and perversion invaded our walls like it was normal. Being a child, it was the only normal I knew, but the funniest thing happens when puberty hits. As a girl, you start your period and step into young womanhood, and something clicks in your head that sexual abuse is real, and not right. The games of touching each other had to stop. This sexual demon had to stop. I had to reclaim my life while I had the chance, but the truth is that even though I stopped participating in the games and touching, that spirit followed me. Depression for me began right at the brinks of puberty. I began to feel unclean, impure, contaminated with the lustful desires of someone who violated and opened that door. You believe you don't have a choice in the matter, so you do what they say, and you keep quiet.

When I would go to school, I was laughed at, not only because of my clothes, but that I was a depressed child who kept to myself because of what was happening to me. When I was in first grade, I went to *Lewis Metropolitan Christian School* in Los Angeles, California. I remember like it was yesterday. Most of the girls would play this game of touching each other. It was about six or seven of us. Everyone would wait until recess when the teachers left out of the classrooms. It would be dark in the room, and each child would take turns going in and laying on top of this one boy for a couple of minutes. I was the lookout most times. The boy, Jeremy, was someone I really liked, and he liked me. One day during recess we went upstairs where no one could see us, and we kissed and touched each other. During class, most of the students were touching each other under the table. I started to see at a very young age that I wasn't alone. If the children in my class knew what touching was, and how to do it, it made me believe that something was happening in their homes, or by a family friend. I did not think much of it until after puberty, and then I understood that this spirit was so real, not only in my life, but others around me. During my teen years, it remained the same, and the teasing and taunting continued until my first suicide attempt at twelve years old when I held a knife to my neck.

I am not the type of person to say, "that was at twelve years old and you're older now, so get over it." I have heard this before many times, and it's a shame because it does not matter if it happened at three or thirty-three. The point is when you do not deal with the issue, it follows you all the days of your life, until you deal with it, or die with it in you. I have said it before, it grows up with you, and if you do not seek professional help and talk about it, it will continue to grow, and depression plays a big part in that.

You ever wonder why some people you meet act a certain way? They could be quiet, loud, or seem like they are *one french fry short of a happy meal*. It does not necessarily mean they were abused, but everything has a root, and they act the way they do based on life experiences. I shied away from hugs because of the sexual abuse. It did not matter if it was a *church pat* or kiss on the cheek, I was not having it. What you could do was back out of my personal space, and dare not look me in the eyes because my story lives there. Thinking about how I used to be, I would constantly look to the ground when spoken to. I don't know when I started doing this, but I was in my mid-twenties still harboring that characteristic. I remember at twenty-six years old I was standing in the hall of the church. I had started learning how to look up from the ground and make eye contact when speaking, even if it was for a brief moment. The pastor said something to me, and I looked towards him. He then said, "do you realize you speak with your eyes?" I have been this way my whole life. I still speak with my eyes to this day, but have learned how to make eye contact and give the other person I am speaking to some respect.

It was not until I started going back to the abuse that I realized how damaged I felt. I was never going to grow from this place if I couldn't accept a hug, a generous embrace from someone who wasn't trying to violate me. I couldn't take in a *three second hug,* even in the church, and that bothered me. It felt like my abusers were coming in all over again for the kill, and because of that the reflection I gave was the persona of being closed off. This may have related to some people that I didn't want to be bothered. *This is far from the truth*. I was a fragile scared girl who held the key to my own chains, and didn't realize it.

This is serious business. There are so many people that grow up with these issues and never say a word because of shame, or it may be that they are scared. Whatever the case may be, I can guarantee that someone around you have experienced sexual abuse, and you don't even know it. In this instance, I am putting on my lipstick and speaking about some of my experiences. Like the old hymn says, *"we shall overcome by the blood of the lamb and the word of our testimony."*

DOES ABUSE APPLY TO YOU? IF SO, HAVE YOU OVERCOME?

4

SWEPT UNDER THE RUG

"Darkness are those little particles of dust hidden away under the rug. Each particle is connected to a name, a place, an incident, an abuse. The only way to see the light is to lift up the rug and sweep out the trash."

Sweeping things under the rug is a tradition passed down by generations to those willing to uphold the mantle. If something happens in the family that would otherwise bring shame and disappointment, you do not mention it to anyone. You do not dare bring it up during dinner or family discussions. Keep it to yourself. The term, for those who may not understand, "swept under the rug", means to keep it a secret as if your life depended on it. You do not literally find a rug, lift it up and sweep it under. It is more a figure of speech. Keep your mouth shut! Don't you dare speak of such things as long as you are part of this family. It's no wonder why so many of us grow up with problems. We are taught at a young age to not deal with it, even if it is killing you.

If you have been abused in any shape, form or fashion and are told to keep silent on the matter, that's the second red flag. The first red flag is the fact that your abuser did this to you, that this act of evil took place. The third red flag is when you tell a parent or guardian and they do nothing about it, or maybe they were the abusers. I declare you better tell it anyway! I was guilty of sweeping it all under the rug for many years as a child and well into my adulthood. This is not healthy. I say to you, even if you are no longer a child and are older like myself, it is okay to start where you are in dealing with it. I recommend, first, forgiving yourself. The *rug* you once swept it under can no longer contain your pain. This *rug* tradition was handed down from generation to generation, but the powerful thing about generational curses and strongholds are that they can be broken, demolished, cast back to where it came from.

Healing must take place. I have been taught this throughout my life, but never applied healing to my everyday life. I am not so sure I knew how. I kept up with the routine of being silent, sweeping the abuse under the rug, and staying committed to the routine of church. This is not a good way to live because one day your past will slap you in the face when you least expect it. At some point, you must deal with the emotional barriers that are weighing you down. Deal with them so that you can fully live the life designed for you to live. Healing is necessary, but sometimes you need guidance.

It is okay to go beyond the four walls of the church and seek professional help. Am I saying that God cannot heal you? No. God can heal you! There have been so many things that God has dealt with me on, brought me out of, walked me through it, and the list goes on and on. So yes, God can heal you, but a person who is dealing with depression must understand that God has already healed you, but because they're dealing with depression, they have to find the tools to learn to walk into their healing and that could be a process.

> *"Everything has a root, but not everyone understands the connection."*

My prayer is that anyone who is afraid to admit it, I'm here to let you know it's okay to be a Christian and admit it. I am at a powerful point in my life where saying it teaches me to walk in my healing. I used to think that by me going to the altar, getting prayer, and falling out prostrate would do it. But I've been learning that when you've experienced depression and anxiety for years, you're going to have to fight when no one is looking and it is a journey. People will not make you happy. I used to think so. People will show you different versions of emotions, which can be mistaken for happiness when around them. You must plant happiness within yourself.

I went to school, got my degrees and started a career. But what I didn't do was deal with my problems. What I didn't do was get to the bottom of why I felt suicidal, why I felt like giving up, and why I felt like I didn't matter anymore. It makes me think about the times when people say, *"all you need is God"*, or *"all you need is a scripture in the word of God"*. This is true as a believer because all you really need is God. But do you know that scripture at some point will not hold power in your life if you don't deal with you. You have to get a hold of the problem or it'll become self-sabotaging and you'll destroy everything around you and not even know it. The last thing you want to do is destroy the greatness in you before you have a chance to see a better outcome.

I was watching an episode of "Iyanla Fix My Life" online one day. Iyanla, a self-empowerment coach was dealing with a married couple and the continuous infidelity they were struggling with. What made this episode most intriguing is that the husband who slept with multiple women outside his marriage was the pastor. His wife, of course, was the first lady. As the story unraveled, Iyanla spoke to the wife separate from the husband. The wife, who was near tears, described how she felt humiliated as a woman and how she was trying to get through to her husband. I continued watching because something struck a chord with me. Iyanla then sat down with the husband and began to dig deep into what was happening. In the beginning, you saw no emotion from the husband, but as the interview continued some things were revealed. This man, who was called by God to lead and help deliver God's people was struggling. His story concluded with the reveal of him being molested as a child, and resulted in what manifested in his life today. Why am I sharing this story with you? It is because everything has a root, but not everyone understands the connection.

The depression I experienced coupled with my sexual struggles and suicidal attempts stemmed from being abused as a child. These things began to manifest into my life when I got older because I did not recognize the trauma in the beginning. I gave it room to grow by not dealing with the problem and it almost cost me my sanity. As for the preacher, because that door of sexual abuse was opened for him as a child, his urges became stronger as an adult, and regardless of who he was, he acted out in what he knew. It did not matter if he had a wife or was a prominent pastor to his congregation. When you sweep things under the rug, not only are you trying to hide the problem, but you are stunting your growth and preventing a greater *you* to shine forward.

WHAT'S UNDER YOUR RUG?

_____

_____

_____

_____

_____

_____

_____

_____

_____

_____

Present

PEOPLE WITH ANXIETY LIVE IN THE PRESENT

5

FORGIVENESS: UNDERSTANDING WHAT HAPPENED

*"Disappointments will try and break you, but I have the power
to change the game. And I will."*

Forgiveness can be very complicated. I would always pride myself on growing and getting past the pain I experienced as a child, but then realized that forgiveness was the most important test, which I failed time and time again. You can forgive someone, and not forgive someone at the same time. Let me explain. If your actions do not line up with your words, then your forgiveness is in vain. You can say, "I forgive this person", but then still have ill feelings towards them. If every time you think of them, you start to feel disgusted by what tore you apart, or the act that took place, you haven't truly forgiven. These are the symptoms I had. Every time my abusers came across my mind, I would get sick to the stomach. Every time I thought about the abuse and incest that happened in my family, I would get nauseous. The pit of my stomach would turn, and I would become a little girl all over again; scared, nervous, afraid. This is not true forgiveness. You are not supposed to continue feeling violated and abused when you forgive. You are supposed to release whatever is making you sick so that you can be free.

> *"I was sitting in the pew becoming
> unfamiliar with my healing."*

Bitterness will suck the living life out of you. I don't want to wake up and see bitterness staring at me in my own reflection. The only way that I could overcome this bitterness, this depression was to admit it; scream it out loud from the mountain top: *No one saved me!* There, I said it. My mind kept repeating itself as I set on the edge of the bed while Jesse pulls his penis out of his pants and masturbates. He looks at me and smiles. I am ashamed. At seven-years-old I am no longer comfortable in my own skin. He continued stroking his penis up and down. The door was closed and locked, and my sister sat on the edge of the bed watching. His grandmother was in the other room sleep. Jesse, forced my little hand to touch it. My sister did nothing. This particular moment happened not long before the actual abuse took place in the back closet, where my seven-year-old body became fragile to touch, and no longer innocent.

The slap in the face for me was when I figured out that I had given my mind, my heart, and my spirit to so many people. Years later, I was still waiting to be saved. I was waiting for someone to open the bedroom door, as I sat on the bed, and save me from the abuse. As I got older, I felt ashamed that I allowed myself to forget my life in Jesus. I felt that he was becoming a stranger because I was too worried about people. So, I followed my heart and took a sabbatical from going to church. This may sound crazy to Christians because fellowship is a necessity to building relationships in Christ, but I was sitting in the pew becoming unfamiliar with my healing. I needed to find my way back to God and quickly lose religion.

I have discovered on this journey that true forgiveness is connected to some major components. The items below are continuing to help me stay out of darkness.

🍂 *Understanding what happened.*

I could not quite put my finger on why things happened the way they did. It took me years to even to get over the fact that it happened. I started to find more understanding in my heart. You must understand that it wasn't your fault, and that God forgives so that you can forgive.

🔖 *Pray.*

Prayer works! I always had trust in prayer being the major key in my survival, but the difference is that I was praying for the wrong things. For example, I used to pray that God would take my life because my suicidal attempts were never successful. This is a good thing that God did not listen to those prayers. Then I would pray just to make it through, which isn't bad. I had to learn that my prayers needed to speak life in the situation and not be so dark. When you are depressed, it can be difficult to really grasp this concept because you do not clearly see the light.

🔖 *Forgive yourself.*

This was my biggest challenge. I had so many memories that I was holding onto, and it was clouding my better judgement. If it is sexual abuse you are dealing with, even as an adult, you must realize that it wasn't your fault. Forgive yourself so that you can be free from those chains. It may not be easy in the beginning, but if you pray and ask for understanding, it will become easier. I know this for a fact.

🔖 *Release those memories.*

The last thing, I believe, is learning to release the pain and hurt of what you have been holding in for so long. It will make you sick to the core, and stop you from living an authentic life. I would always give it to God, then take it back unknowingly. When I discovered what I was doing I began opening up more, and allowing those things that were holding me back to be released. I am not perfect, and am still working on myself, but the beauty in it is that I am starting to live a little freer than before because of the release.

Unforgiveness caused me to be depressed and no one knew it. I walked around with a smile on my face, but inside I was hurting. I mastered the art of putting on a façade. I hid behind my smile. I allowed memories of the past to keep me internally stagnant, and it was just a matter of time before I exploded. Depression left me mentally unstable, and I began to believe those lies all over again that I was ugly, nobody loved me and that "God didn't bless people like me". Someone in the church actually said those words to my face, and I continued hearing those words years later. Do not let yourself get so depressed that you become unrecognizable to your own image in the mirror. Seek help at the first sign of depression by praying and reaching out.

When I was in undergrad, my Creative Writing teacher gave all the students an exercise. We had to write out ten forgiveness's on a sheet of paper so that we can clear our minds to being vulnerable as we write. Although we did not have to turn it in, I often look at my list. Surprisingly, when I reference it, I no longer feel shame.

Here are a couple of my 10 forgiveness's:

1. *I forgive you dad for not being there when I needed you.*

If men are reading this book, I would say to you: *please, be there for your children because either way it will have an impact on their lives.* I would say this to the men because we become a reflection of what they sow into us, sometimes unknowingly. I used to despise hearing the church say to people, "Let God Be Your Father". I would get irritated because I did not understand the concept of allowing someone to be your father, and you couldn't even see them. It wasn't until it clicked spiritually for me. I was going through so much, feeling depressed and stressed out. I remember crying myself to sleep, like I did many nights, and in the midst of my tears it felt as if the arms of God reached down and wrapped me up. It really felt as if arms were holding me, and I knew that I was home alone. I woke up the next day feeling peace and knew without a shadow of a doubt that God was my father, my comforter, my source of strength. That experience really helped to nurture my forgiveness when it came to not having my father in my life.

2. *I forgive the girl in junior high who teased and taunted me until everyone laughed.*

It is never easy for a child to experience being bullied. It causes major emotional and mental instability in that child, not to mention, most children will grow up either wanting revenge or wanting to take their own lives. I was at the end of both spectrums: wanting to die and wanting them to feel what I felt when they teased me. I remember writing a letter on Facebook to one of the girls that teased me in junior high. Twenty years later, I reached out to her apologizing for rejecting her when she reached out to me a few years back. I also let her know that my reason for doing so was because she bullied me in junior high and it made me feel worthless. I apologized for holding the little girl she was to the grown woman she had become. I never got a response though it showed she read it, and I wasn't expecting one, but it taught me *true forgiveness*. I had to release her mentally so that I could move on and not be afraid of relationships. I could not continue holding this against her if I wanted to heal.

WHAT ARE YOUR TEN FORGIVENESS'S?

1.
_____

2.
_____

3.
_____

4.
_____

5.
_____

6.
_____

7.

_____

8.

_____

9.

_____

10.

_____

WHO DO YOU NEED TO FORGIVE? HAVE YOU FORGIVEN YOURSELF?

6

WHO TO TRUST?

"Many are dealing with trust issues and do not even realize it. The beauty of having trust issues is that you have an opportunity to deal with you before you can deal with anyone else."

hen dealing with depression it is very difficult to trust anyone. Most people cannot understand the emotional damage behind trust, and what may cause a person to have those issues. I knew that I did not trust anyone. The mere fact that all my relationships growing up led to everyone leaving caused me to not trust anyone. Just like everything else, I had to go back and find what triggered my lack of trust. *There was a method to my madness*, as the saying goes. There were reasons why I did not know how to love, live, be free or build strong relationships. I did not have good examples growing up, therefore I didn't know the first thing to becoming better. These are the examples that I had as a child:

- *Siblings*: No one talked to each other, or got along. There was always fighting and arguing, and the abuse was heavy. Being the baby, I felt like they did not care to be my sisters because all they did was talk about me, make me cry and pushed me to attempt *suicide*.

- *Mother:* I used to feel abandoned, being that we were constantly homeless, and I was on the street at an early age. I did not think my mother loved me, and I carried those feelings for many years. It was not until I got a little older and wiser that I began to forgive my mother for what she did not know. But before that point in my life, I carried *abandonment* like a badge of honor.

🐾 *Father:* I was never able to have a relationship with my father. He was a very abusive man to all of us. I remember getting slapped by him because my voice was too low and he wanted me to speak up. I remember him making my mother stop the car in the middle of the street by hitting her so that he could reach in the back to lash my sisters and I with his belt. I remember running up to him at three years old at my grandmother's house and my mother grabbing me while she whispered, "don't you ever run up to that man again." She was afraid of him. He died when I was fourteen and my image of *trusting* men was tainted.

🐾 *Friends:* I was so quiet in school, but managed to make a couple friends, at least I thought they were. In grade school, they would taunt and tease me for my image and what I didn't have. I was *bullied* and often forced into the bathroom stall so that they could jump me.

🐾 *Church:* This was my saving grace. At the age of sixteen, I joined a small Baptist church. It was the first time that I felt like I belonged somewhere even though my personal life got more difficult. Due to my previous examples, I did not know how to have a proper relationship, so I *struggled* in church and they did not know how to handle it. I remained suicidal singing in the choir and being part of the Youth and Young Adult Ministry.

The reason why I listed the above examples is because sometimes you have to go back and find out why your trust is barren. You have to look at your examples growing up and see if you can pinpoint where these traits came from so that you can change them. For some people, you may have had a good childhood but feel you can't trust anyone because of one incident. Go to that place and figure it out. For others, your upbringing may be the key you need to overcome. Take some time to see your past relationships in your childhood so that you can adjust what you need to move forward. In the below exercise, you have an opportunity to go back in time and discover where your trust became stagnant. You can follow my example above, if it deals with your upbringing, or just write what comes to your heart.

List examples of why it is difficult for you to trust:

  _____

_____

_____

_____

  _____

_____

_____

_____

  _____

_____

ARE YOU EXPERIENCING TRUST ISSUES? WHERE DO THEY STEM FROM? HOW ARE YOU OVERCOMING THEM?

_____

_____

_____

_____

_____

_____

_____

_____

7

BECOMING HEALTHY

"I had to clip those wings of being a victim and fall from it,
but instead I flew."

This is easier said than done. At least it was for me because I did not know the first steps to a healthier life. When I talk about becoming healthy, I am basically referring to working on your *mental, spiritual and emotional* well-being. There were times I felt like I was going insane because I did not know how to handle all the situations coming my way. I had to be very careful because although suicide was not an option, at certain points, I tried it. I tried talking to pastors, but would get sent off with a scripture and no spiritual guidance. I tried speaking to friends, but of course they did not know how to deal with the load I was carrying. It was not until undergrad at San Francisco State University that I had my first professional counseling session.

During my session, we talked about what I was dealing with. It was at this point that I realized I had been carrying childhood trauma and I was pushing thirty-years-old. Just like the saying goes, "age ain't nothing but a number". You could be fifty and still carry the load of your past on your shoulders. What kind of life is that? We also talked about the sexual abuse and for the first time in my life I felt like someone was listening to me. The counselor mentioned that she was going to report the abuse to (CPS) Child Protective Services even though I was grown. Her reasoning was because it happened when I was a child and this person may still be around children. I felt relieved because someone was finally saving me from sitting on the edge of the bed as the abuse took place, not in a literal sense, but mentally the chains were falling. It's hard to explain, but someone was finally caring about my well-being and actually doing something about it. I was tired of screaming inside and no one listening. It got so bad for me that I learned how to block out my screams from within and at some point, I couldn't hear the noise. It was not easy, but I had to begin focusing on those screams, hoping they would lead me to the little girl who held her own healing, and I could follow the echoes. Part of my therapy session included going back to those memories that haunted me.

> *"Becoming healthy is more than just physical, it's dealing with those voices filling you up with lifeless thoughts."*

There was this one time in my life when my then god-sister, whom I adored, dropped me off at the house I was living in. I quickly got out of the car so that she wouldn't get out to walk me, but she got out anyway. As we walked up to the door, my heart felt like it was about to drop out of my chest. I did not want her to see what was happening behind that door, so I avoided inviting her in. *Behind that door was death.* When you first walked in, there was trash throughout the living room and clothes everywhere. There was a stench that smelled like old moth balls and mildew, a glass jar filled with tears and another suicide attempt. I was barely sixteen. Her facial expressions told me she knew something was going on, but she never said much about it. This is just one of many experiences I had, but never dealt with what was going on inside of my head. Becoming healthy is more than just physical, it's dealing with those voices filling you up with lifeless thoughts: "you don't deserve to be here", "no one cares about you", "she'll leave you like they all have", "don't bother dreaming, you're dead anyways". Those thoughts will kill you mentally as they did me, but there was something deeply rooted in my heart that kept pulling me out of darkness.

There was another experience when I tried to stay at my sister's house because I was homeless. My sister did not speak to me, neither did she want me at her house. I was tired of staying on the streets, here and there, and thought that maybe my sister would take me in. I was wrong. I remember coming into her house in Inglewood, California right down the street from Centinela Park. My sister, her husband and children, though the kids had no say so in the matter, would stay out all day until one o'clock in the morning. When they finally arrived home, I would be sitting on the porch waiting patiently. They would get out the car, go inside and never check to see if I was okay. They would do things like this constantly to make me feel uncomfortable, and they succeeded until I could no longer go back there. Besides, I wasn't their responsibility. I was only their sister. I learned to walk the streets, parks and neighborhoods all day because I had nowhere else to go. These are memories I had to revisit on my self-discovery journey. It may not seem like much to some, but those experiences caused me to feel unwanted by my own flesh and blood.

I continued counseling during undergrad and even started to see a personal therapist after graduation. This was the beginning steps of becoming healthy, and I knew it was going to be a long road, but it was a step in the right direction. I constantly had to go back to the little girl inside of me and comfort her, as well as grow her. Becoming healthy also includes assessing your life as a child and seeing where you are now. There were times when I would write down on a sheet of paper how I felt as a *little girl*, and compare it with how I feel as a grown woman *(big girl)*. This was a great way for me to notice all the feelings that were being conjured up as an adult did not have room to linger in my present or future. I only felt those emotions because I was allowing myself to remember without being healed. When I see the contrast between the two, it pushes me to continue fighting through it all. On the next page, I have listed my example exercise on how I separated the two during my healing process.

Big Girl/Little Girl Defined:

Little Girl	*Big Girl*
Been hurt	Takes hurt and dreams BIG
Been abused	FIGHTS to end abuse and speaks truth
Been forgotten	Does not understand the word NO
Been ignored	Gravitates to HAPPINESS
Been neglected by family	Celebrates herself
Hides in a corner, *alone*	Shouts to the world that she is somebody!
Writes her pain	Writes her vision
Hard for her to let go	Let's go of the past and moves on

Here is your opportunity to define the *little girl or boy* inside of you. Use the left side of this chart to begin understanding what you are still holding onto, so that there can be a difference in how the roots of those strongholds work. Then use the right side of the chart to see how far you have come.

Little Girl (or Boy)	*Big Girl (or Boy)*

WHAT STEPS ARE YOU TAKING TO BECOME HEALTHY?

_____

_____

_____

_____

_____

_____

_____

_____

8

WHAT IS THE ENEMY SCARED OF?

"There is a major shift in a person's life when they realize that the enemy is more afraid of them than they think."

ave you ever thought about why you're experiencing depression, anxiety or stress more than you should? Or why it seems like you've fallen into a hole and there is no one around to help pull you out? I once heard someone say that the life you're experiencing is based on the series of choices you've made overtime. We allow ourselves to stay committed to situations that aren't good, and wonder why we get depressed. I can't stress how many times I would keep holding onto the past when it was trying to let me go. I kept it here. I allowed those memories to take up residence in my life. Why is that? It is because most of us do not know how to let go of the past. I would always sit at home and get depressed because I was lonely. I felt that no one wanted to be around me due to my past experiences. I was conditioned to think that I was worthless. I was taught that I wouldn't become anything and no one wanted me.

> *"I began asking questions so that I could better understand who I am."*

Although I understand it wasn't my fault, and definitely not yours, I gave depression a place to take a shower, a bed to sleep in and cover to keep warm. Just like allowing family to come and stay with you for a short period, it can be hard to get them out of your house. Once I gave depression residence, it got stronger, which in return made me feel weaker. This opens the door for depression to take priority over your life, and for all the negative things to begin training your mind. When the damage is released in you, you lose the positive function you need to fight. I noticed the change in me when I was physically here but my spirit wasn't. I had been disconnected and it left me vulnerable and afraid. At some point, I started to learn how to treat myself. I learned that there are several things I can do to lift myself up. It all starts in the mind, and as long as there was life left in me, I was going to fight. What you think about yourself determines how you feel, but when you realize that you are more powerful than you think, the *shift* will happen.

I define the *shift* as:

> /shift/
>
> *a moment when you recognize your potential in the midst of your despair.*

You can be at your lowest point in life and still experience a *shift*. Your mindset begins to change and you see much clearer. When my *shift* happened, I began asking questions so that I could better understand who I am. The questions I asked myself put me in a position for restoration. I needed to be restored. I knew that I couldn't keep living my life this way. A dear friend once told me that a person won't change their situation, even if it's unhealthy, until it hurts enough. You can be experiencing the worst years of your life, but until you make it up in your mind, you'll continue reliving the past. I had to decide on what I wanted in life, and I knew that these situations were temporary because I said so. When you finally *say so,* you take authority over your life.

In 2007, I moved from Sacramento, California back to Los Angeles for a period of three months during the summer. While I was experiencing homelessness and instability once again, staying with a friend, which I understand now is not always good, I began to learn more about myself. I struggled with independency because that little girl inside of me was fighting for support, love, understanding. During that time, relationships were broken, some of which I cried because it was unexpected. I was heartbroken, but determined to find my way out of that mess. I have talked about it before, but this was the time I slept on a park slide in Centinela Park in Inglewood, California. It was not easy and I felt abandoned, but there was no turning back. In July, I moved to a little town called Antioch, California. It was then I fought harder than I ever have to begin taking authority over my life. I still experienced pressure and setbacks but I could no longer give up. The transitions with relationships shifted me to become selfish. I had to learn how to first focus on what I wanted, which was hard in the beginning because I was always concerned about everyone else around me. I eventually learned that I was just as important as the next person, and deserved every bit of happiness. It is amazing how life begins to line up when you put yourself first. Life changed for me and I began to feel good about my choices. Below, I share some of my tips that helped me refocus, and believe it or not, I have to revisit these tips when I need it.

Tip 1 Allow yourself to *shift* even when it feels unnatural and uncomfortable. I moved out of my comfort zone, or hometown of Los Angeles, California because I was never comfortable there to begin with.

Tip 2 Except what is so that you can get excited about what is to come. I excepted the severed relationships from my past, though I believed we would be friends or sisters forever.

Tip 3 Focus on one goal and accomplish it. I quickly began working on my second book, and finally completed and released it in 2010. This built momentum for me to complete another goal on my list.

Tip 4 Release your tears when you need to. I had to learn that tears are healthy because when you hold them in, you don't release what you need to.

Face it. *Shifting* will bring about many emotions and honestly, it does not always feel good. But what I have learned is that when you *shift*, you grow. I went through a purging season in my life after I moved. I tried reaching out to people that I was the closest to in Los Angeles, but realized they chose to eliminate me from their lives. It was hard, but I had to literally *purge my emotions, shed my tears, talk to someone about it, and move on*. I said a prayer to send them well wishes, and moved on. I began to be more purposeful about what I wanted in my life, and focused more on my intentions, opposed to what happened before the *shift*. Please remember that throughout all of life's unexpected circumstances, you are stronger than you think. The enemy is afraid you'll accomplish what's inside of you.

The greatest discovery you can unfold is understanding your purpose in life. Write it down on a sheet of paper or in a journal and meditate on it. If you can't figure out what it is, seek your purpose through prayer. To begin, you can ask yourself these questions that have helped me on the next page.

Who am I that the enemy keeps picking on me?

🐾 _____

_____

_____

_____

Why does the enemy want to destroy my life?

🐾 _____

_____

_____

_____

Why do I continue to have bad thoughts about myself?

🐾 _____

_____

_____

_____

Why am I having thoughts of suicide? Or why can't I get over a specific situation?

🐾 _____

_____

_____

_____

ADDITIONAL NOTES...

Five Stages to Dealing with Depression

As we continue forward with this book, I want to begin discussing the five most important stages that can help when dealing with depression. Of course, there are more stages, some of which I continue to discuss in prospective chapters. The most important thing in this model is to discover what works for you. These below are a perfect way to begin the journey of overcoming depression.

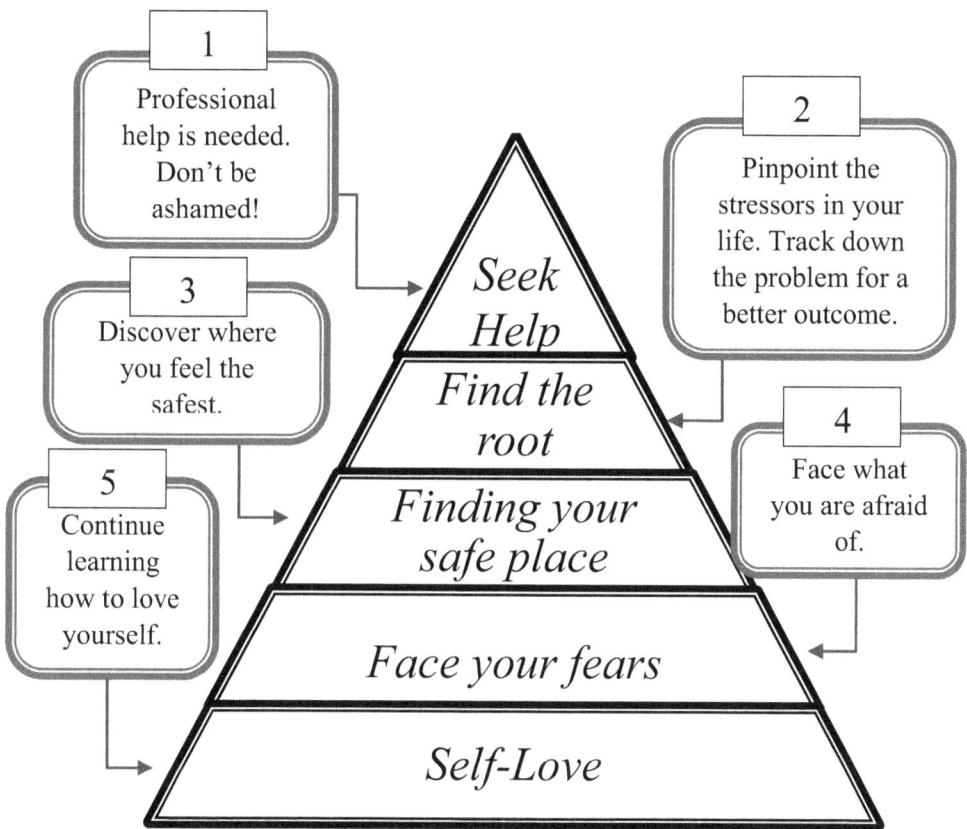

1
Professional help is needed. Don't be ashamed!

2
Pinpoint the stressors in your life. Track down the problem for a better outcome.

3
Discover where you feel the safest.

4
Face what you are afraid of.

5
Continue learning how to love yourself.

Seek Help

Find the root

Finding your safe place

Face your fears

Self-Love

THE FUTURE

HAPPY PEOPLE LIVE IN THE FUTURE

9

GRATITUDE JOURNAL

*"Gratefulness only comes to those who seek it. It is only when you
decide to look towards the light that you'll come out of darkness."*

Being grateful is the most therapeutic way to climb out of depression. I was always grateful for something, but it was never enough to change my mindset. I would wake up in the morning and say, "God, thank you for this day", but as the day went on I allowed depression to overwhelm me. It is okay to be grateful for your day. As a matter of fact, that is a good starting point to being grateful. The problem is, I stayed right there. I never graduated from, "God, I thank you for this day", and my thoughts never changed. One day, I was journaling how my day went, and how I felt heaviness hovering over me. I began to see those words becoming true in my life. The more I wrote about darkness, the heavily it appeared in some shape, form or fashion. When you release unhealthy thoughts into the atmosphere, you are basically saying, "come back to me fully grown" as if it were a boomerang. And it will. It'll come back in a different form and you'll wonder why you are going through that situation.

> *"Your most powerful seed are your
> words."*

Just like previous chapters, I had to change the way I released things into the atmosphere. I understand that there is a return on words, and if you are not careful, they will manifest like wolves in sheep clothing. You'll think something is good for you until you get burned. About seven years ago, my pastor said to me during a meeting, *"Your most powerful seed are your words."* I believed it then, and I believe it now. What I speak has power to form, so I needed to be careful on what I said about myself. I continued journaling and soon I was saying things like, "I'm grateful for my job" or "I am grateful for the roof over my head". The more I said it, the more I became appreciative for the things I did have. This caused me to create a gratitude journal where I listed things I am grateful for. It doesn't have to be deep. You do not have to write in paragraph form, or do spellcheck. You just write what you are grateful for as it comes to you.

I noticed my mood would change, and material things were less important to me. It did not matter if I had the latest Apple Watch or drove a BMW. What mattered is that after all the mental damage I allowed myself to fall in, God still kept me. I was no longer dancing with the devil, and that gave me peace. When your mood changes, your mindset changes and you become more powerful in your life. This was a great start of my transition from dealing with the past and allowing those memories to haunt me in my own skin. It is a scary thing to feel like your body is a cemetery where the bones of your past lay rampant, contaminated by your own breath. When you come out of something so mentally deep, it becomes an awakening. *Gratefulness* added to this process. The more I wrote it, it became easier to speak it, and as I spoke it, others started to see the change.

Gratitude journals become your message. It gains purpose and momentum in your life because you are finding gratitude in everything around you. It's like a boomerang; eventually it comes back to you. It may not be in the form you would expect, but the gratitude of others will help to transform your life. You will find yourself right amid acts of kindness, and individuals assigned to your life. I have experienced this on a major level, and some of the people I have never met a day in my life. I had experiences where I was grateful for my education but did not know how tuition was going to get paid. Then I would receive a check in the mail towards my education from someone across the country. I would be grateful for what little food I did have, and someone would ring my doorbell with bags of groceries because they thought of me. I would be grateful for my car and have a quarter tank of gas, then someone would slip a $20 bill in my hand. Before I purchased a car, I would show gratefulness for my legs as I walked to work, and someone I knew would pull right beside me offering a ride. You get what I'm saying? The more grateful you become, the more you allow all good to find you.

There's a difference in your mindset when gratefulness becomes your identical twin. I haven't always been this way, but it is an amazing feeling to be grateful for what is yet to come. I find it an honor to face opposition and still look towards the future. Most people, like myself, will face trials and allow depression to get the best of them. This is why you have to teach yourself to *see* beyond, allowing gratefulness to infiltrate your heart, mind and soul. I must constantly tell myself, "you are chosen and deserve to be here." Here is an example of my gratitude journal:

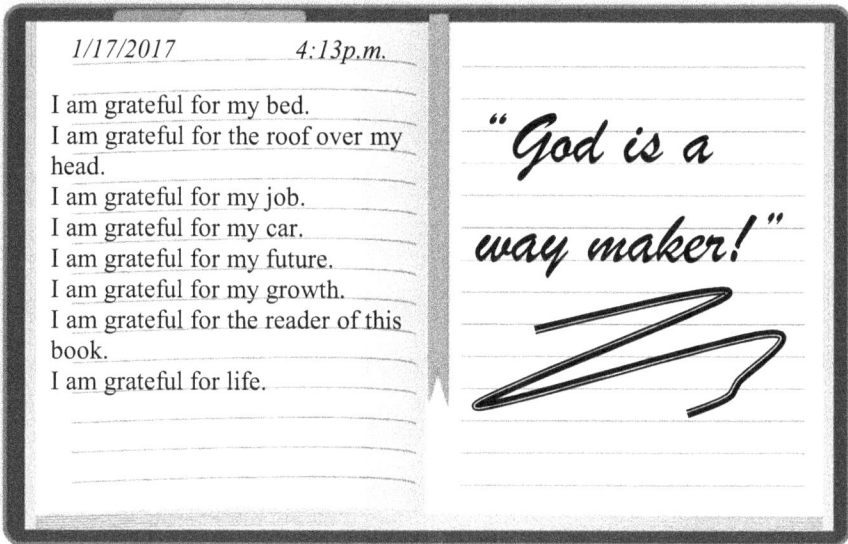

1/17/2017	4:13p.m.

I am grateful for my bed.
I am grateful for the roof over my head.
I am grateful for my job.
I am grateful for my car.
I am grateful for my future.
I am grateful for my growth.
I am grateful for the reader of this book.
I am grateful for life.

"God is a way maker!"

Like I stated before, it does not have to be deep or thoroughly written out. You just briefly write what comes to your mind. It is okay if you repeat things everyday because what it does is create a form of positive repetition in your mind, thus changing your outcome. You will be amazed at how you feel about yourself, and how others will begin to gravitate towards you.

ARE YOU KEEPING A GRATITUDE JOURNAL? NAME 10 THINGS YOU ARE GRATEFUL FOR?

1.

2.

3.

4.

5.

6.

7.

8.

9.

10.

10

TRANSFORMING YOUR WALLS INTO DOORS

"Eventually they are no longer here. We are no longer here. We soon vanish. That's why we must live."

*T*he most important moment is when I learned to speak up for myself. People did not like it. I lost "friends" because of it. It is amazing how people want you to stay the victim but as soon as you reach higher than yourself and speak up, they'll have something to say. Regardless, they'll always have something to say.

Lisa Nichols, self-empowerment speaker and coach once said during an interview, "the world is following your example on how to treat you." This was an *ah-ha* moment for me because I sincerely believe that a lot of my depression dealt with wanting the acceptance of others, wanting to be remembered and not forgotten, wanting people to love me and reach out for me. This was desolate in my childhood, which made me crave it. One thing about depression is that it stems from something. I had to look back at my life and find out why I would get so depressed at certain points. I discovered that depression would creep in around the holidays, which also happened to be the time leading to my birthday. When the holidays would come, this mask of sadness would shadow over me. I would begin to remember all the holidays we never celebrated as a family. I could not remember one birthday that I celebrated with my family, hearing the song "happy birthday" illuminate the atmosphere. I would remember these moments and begin to feel like my existence did not matter. Eventually, I would carry all those emotions into the new year not knowing that I was creating this path of depression to follow me all the days of my life.

What I am finding out is that people around me and people that I meet the first time are accepting the offer I'm giving them on how to treat me. What I'm saying is when a person goes through depression, they sink into themselves; they feel alone, abandoned, and they feel like no one cares. For me, I would hide into myself not wanting to be around other people, then worry about why no one is reciprocating love back to me. The mask of depression began to hover over my life. I gave them the approval to treat me this way unknowingly. I gave them the approval because I wasn't tending to myself. I began to understand that they are just reflecting what I am to myself. How are you treating yourself? How are you showing your soul to the world?

> *"Transform your memories into lessons and focus on where you're headed, instead of where you have been."*

When it came to my education, I always felt like I could accomplish this dream, but because I had dropped out so many times, I pulled further from this goal. I knew that I wanted to promote higher education and help students to see past their circumstances, but in order to do this I had to change what I was putting out in the universe. I had to reverse my failed attempts and try again. That's all you can do is try again, but this time make it your business to see it to the end. You have a right to accomplish that thing which you set out to do. This is to be said with every area of your life. Begin to weed through those areas that are prohibiting your goals from flourishing and pull them up at the roots.

Family was my number one stress trigger, and because I finally recognized this, I pulled myself out of the equation. I separated myself from the negativity to give myself a chance to change, and to see what I was capable of in a different setting. I shutdown holding onto unhealthy friendships so that I could experience the true meaning of friendship. I found myself wanting more, becoming more and busting through those walls of opposition.

This realization was so powerful in my life. I came to a crossroad and had to choose the path I wanted to walk. I had to transform my memories into lessons and focus on where I am headed instead of where I have been. The best way to transform your walls into doors is to reassess your life. Write down everything that you feel is holding you back. Write down anything you are holding inside of you. Write down your triggers of what makes you depressed. Talk to a trusted friend. Make an appointment with a counselor. It is okay to seek professional help. Below is an example of how I wrote things down that was hindering me. This is just one example that triggered most of my depression, which I carried into my adulthood. When I thought of the word *family,* these three feelings immediately came to mind.

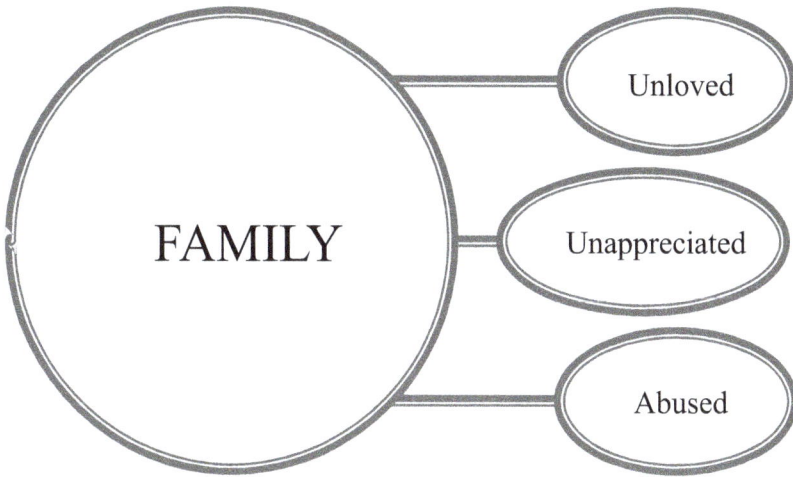

Take a moment in the exercise below to list some of the main causes for your depression. For each cluster, write the three immediate emotions you feel.

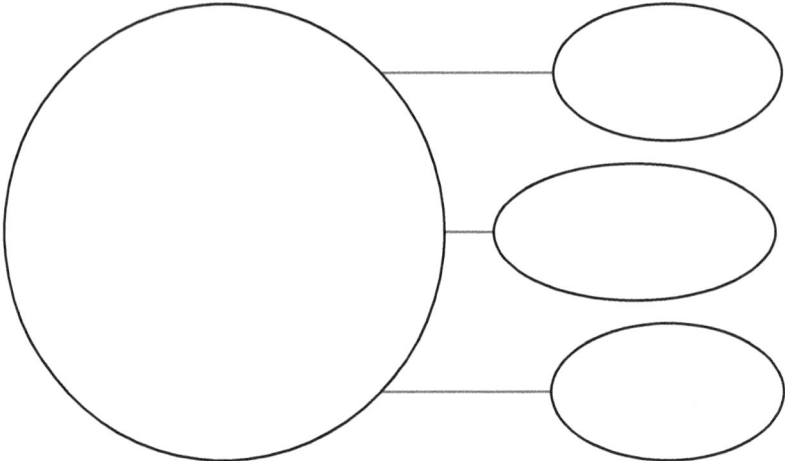

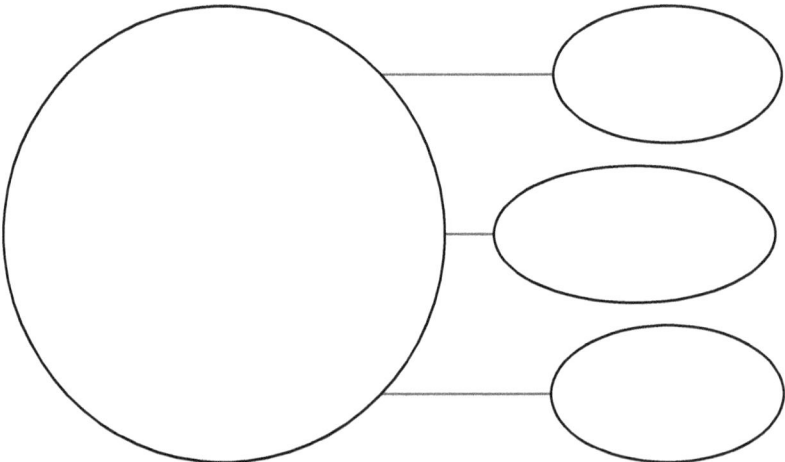

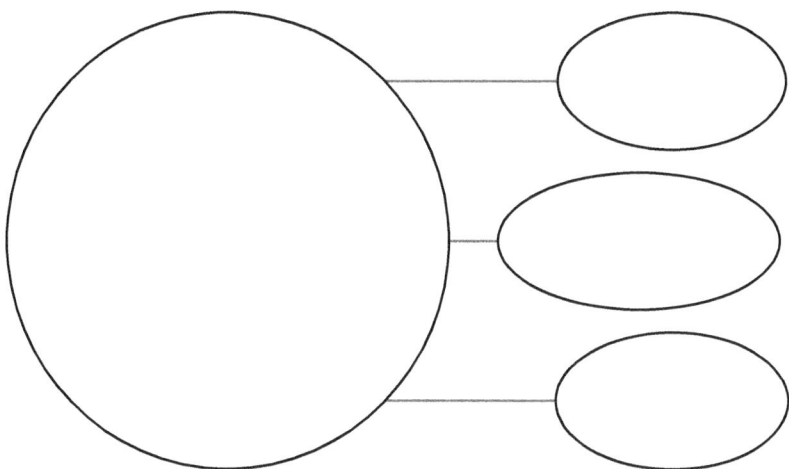

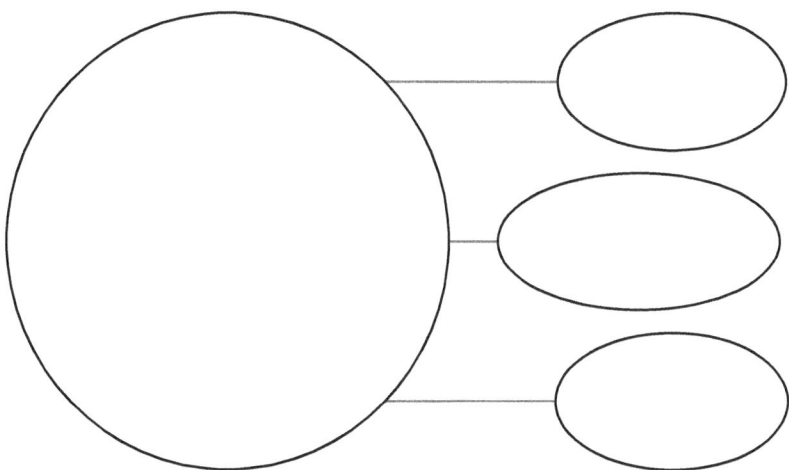

WHAT BRICK WALLS HAVE YOU BUSTED DOWN? EDUCATION? CAREER?
SPIRITUAL? FRIENDSHIPS? FAMILY? HOW HAVE YOU DONE SO?

_____

_____

_____

_____

_____

_____

_____

_____

11

SPEAK INTO YOUR FUTURE

*"I challenge change to build a mountain in front of me
and watch as I climb it."*

You have to replace your limitations with possibilities by speaking into your future. Once you have gone through your past and discovered the key things that ignites your depression, and have dealt with those issues, continue speaking life into yourself. Start in the beginning when you're feeling down and out. Take pride in the fact that what you went through did not kill you, or weaken your outcome. It has made you stronger. If you have gotten this far in the book, I believe you are that much closer to overcoming depression. You may have struggled in certain areas of your life, but make today count by trusting you got this.

> *"I called all those things to me and
> expected them to show up in my life."*

I used to wait on people all the time because I always thought they had it better. If I could just get their attention and follow in their footsteps my life would be that much greater. *Boy, was I wrong!* There were certain times in my life when people would come up to me and say, "You inspire me," or "I'm trying to be like you". I would always look at this person and try to see what they see. The fact is when you are depressed you avoid seeing beauty. I blinded myself from beauty because I was focused on the negative. When I finally began to see what others saw in me, it was like a whole new person appeared. I started seeing myself in the future living a successful life, and reminded myself that whatever trials come my way, I would most definitely get through it. In this moment of actualization, I wrote letters to myself and spoke positive affirmations into the atmosphere. Things like: "You are beautiful!" or "You're going to do great things!" or "You are a manifestation of greatness."

Speaking positive affirmations allowed me to witness a better present. I was able to focus on what was a priority in my life and get things done. I went back to school and received two degrees, studied in England for a year and traveled throughout Europe on a scholarship. If I would have stayed in the depressed mindset, I would have never experienced that type of glory in my life because I would have never applied myself. I called all those things to me and expected them to show up in my life. Speaking into your future is part of the law of attraction. Whatever you think about yourself, you will become. Whatever you want in life, you will receive. I always thought negative about myself because I did not know any other way of thinking. It constantly brought sadness into my life, and everyday was like a funeral. As I began thinking about the positive things I wanted in my life and applied myself, I became more grateful even when storms hit.

I have dealt with many battles in my life, as we all have. During those times, I would journal how I felt about myself, and soon opposed those negative thoughts with positive declarations. These are some of the things I felt about myself on the following page:

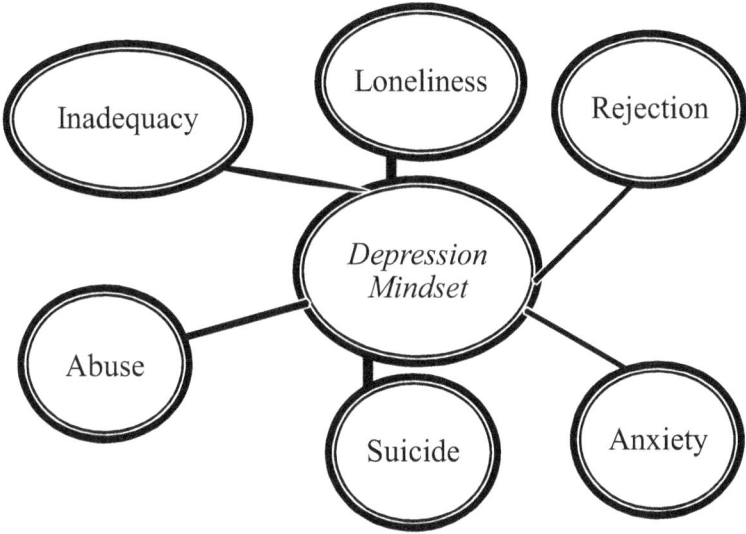

As I started speaking into my future, I changed my thought process, and continually do it on a daily basis. This is what it looks like now that I have a better understanding. This mindset change is a daily battle, but the payoff is great. Take a look on the next page to see what a greatness mindset looks like.

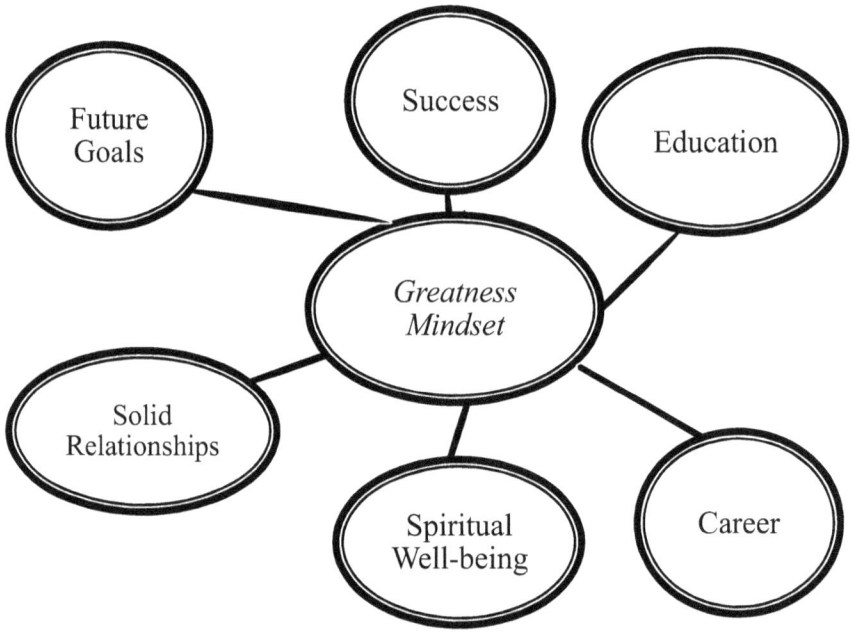

Quit burying yourself before you have an opportunity to live. Stop mentally calling death into your life and get up! Your life is precious, and if you have never heard those words, say it to yourself. Be accountable for you, and others will follow your footsteps. I do not live a perfect life. I have my ups and downs, but am learning to cast depression out of my life every time I feel it trying to creep its way in. I have no vacancy for it, only positive goals I look forward to accomplishing. What are you speaking into yourself? Become present in those thoughts of greatness and watch how your life will change.

WHAT DOES YOUR FUTURE LOOK LIKE?

12

SOCIAL RELATIONSHIPS

"I am remarkably inspired so much that I pushed myself off the cliff of loneliness into a life of possibility."

A nother way, I am constantly learning as well, to change the depression you may be experiencing is to get out more. This was difficult for me because I was never a social butterfly. As a matter of fact, I am an introvert and can only experience so many people at once. Many people are like this, but that doesn't mean you should be content with being alone. You may be thinking, "what does social relationships have to do with depression?" I have an answer based on my experience. When you are depressed, you keep your distance away from people, places and friendships. You always have an excuse as to why you can't do something, or go somewhere. You start feeling bad about yourself, and when the phone rings you send it to voicemail. I am guilty of this. I have done these things far too many times in my life that it became a routine. When this becomes repetitious in your life it can be hard to break.

> *"Stop putting expectations on people because if your expectations aren't met, it'll set you back."*

Here are some lessons I have learned:

- People do not want to be around depressed people. *Remember, moods can transfer.*

- People can sometimes say the things you want to hear out of convenience. For example, "*let me know if you need anything.*"

- People have their own problems to deal with. *We are all dealing with something at some point in our lives.*

- God will send the right people your way to help you through your ordeal. *Someone is always watching even when you don't realize.*

These lessons taught me to stop putting expectations on people because if your expectations aren't met, it will set you back. Your focus should be on you, like their focus is on them. You will begin to do more for yourself, and those people will then gravitate to you. I also learned that it becomes easier to socialize with people because you removed the restraints. You have opened the door to growth, and regardless if you see it or not, people do recognize it.

I do want to mention that this is a daily process for me because I have always been a loner. Being the youngest of a dysfunctional non-communicative family pushed me into loneliness. The most important thing is that I learned how to do things by myself without the expectation of someone being there. If you are feeling like you struggle in this area, try doing some of these things below that helped me, and continues to help me daily.

- *Go to a matinee movie*: On a Saturday afternoon, I would go and see a movie by myself. In the beginning, I wished I had company, but after while it started to feel good, and there were other movie goers sitting alone.

- *Take a long walk in the park*: Walks are calming, and a great way to release some tension.

- *Sit at a coffee shop and write*: This is one of my favorite things to do. It allows me to enjoy a cup of coffee, and follow through on my dreams and goals by writing them down.

- *Spark up a conversation with a stranger*: I always get nervous doing this, but have learned to just say hello when I'm out. You'll be amazed at the conversations that are waiting for you.

- *Join a group at your local church*: Being part of a singles ministry, or group in the church will allow you to meet new people. I have met some great individuals by doing this.

- *Volunteer*: There are many volunteer opportunities to be part of, especially during the holidays. I remember volunteering at my church during the Thanksgiving Food Drive where we gave free dinner plates to the community. This gave me a sense of belonging, and helped those who were less fortunate.

- *Turn off the TV and meditate*: I rarely watch television, so this is not a difficult thing for me to do. I can sit on my bed with my journal and meditate on my future, allowing all the positive vibes to manifest in my life.

What are some things you do to come out of darkness and be more social?

- _____

- _____

- _____

13

FINDING PURPOSE

"You have to fall in love with who you are becoming, and release the person that is destroying you."

People want to have meaning for their purpose in life. They want to feel like they belong and are needed by someone. As a person who has experienced depression, I know that you don't fully understand who you are. Everyone goes through dark times in their lives, whether they show it or not, but everyone doesn't experience depression on a major level. Why is that? I have come to find that knowing who you are plays a role in your mental stability. We all have a God-ordained purpose, but many are not quite sure on what that is. We tend to get confused on thinking that our talent is our purpose, when for some, that could be far from the truth. For others, the talents God gave them is a direct connection to their purpose. I struggled with this for many years. I was always seeking for that power in my life where I knew it was a connection to my purpose. With many failed attempts, seeking other like-minded women for guidance, I have come to realize that what God has for me it is for me, and most importantly, it is already inside of me. That was my biggest problem. I continued searching in everyone else for my purpose hoping that they would give me hope in myself. At some point, people cannot do that for you. You have to learn to find the hope in yourself.

"You are learning how to recover yourself from the trauma you've experienced and held inside of you for too long."

Finding your purpose will give you more perspective in life, and believe it or not, it will help you become more mentally stable. It's hard to explain, but *you have to fall in love with who you are becoming, and release the person that is destroying you.* What I mean is, you must discover all the great aspects of your life and begin to walk towards it. Release that person in you that constantly gets depressed. I had to remind myself that I am more capable of doing great things than I thought. I would repeatedly tell myself, while looking in the mirror, that purpose lies in me and I was meant to be somebody. You, my dear, were designed to be somebody!

Being a writer is one of the greatest gifts that God could have ever given me. Writing has helped me to work out my thoughts on paper when I felt no one was listening. It has helped me to write the depression out of me so that I could see it for what it was; *a negative spirit trying to keep me from knowing who I am.* Find out your purpose in life by first discovering the gifts and talents God gave you. What do you enjoy doing in your life? If you were given an opportunity to do that with minimum pay, then you're on the right track to finding your purpose. If it is something opposite from what you are talented in, then begin nurturing that passion. The most important thing is to pray and ask God to lead you into purpose. Trust me, it works. I don't want to get deep, but it is a spiritual journey. You are learning how to recover yourself from the trauma you've experienced and held inside of you for too long. You are learning that you are worth being here, and the only one that can validate your existence is you. You are learning that it takes a whole lot of courage and strength to release the past. You are learning that this journey is allowing those things to die in you to experience all the goodness your life has to offer, and some do not make it. Most people will die with secrets, heartache, pain, dreams and goals still in them. This is why they say that the graveyard is the richest, wealthiest place in this world. It is also a place where the mourning never stops because most people will die with secrets still in their hearts. Do you want that for yourself? If not, you still have time to turn things around.

My question to you is: How long have you and God been friends? I heard a spiritual counselor say this to a stage four cancer patient. His response, "for a very long time". I have learned that my relationship with God, regardless if I feel like I have fallen, is the best relationship I could ever ask for. *He* knows my weakness and what I need to work on, and if I understand my worth, he'll continue to reveal himself to me. We live in a world where we cannot possibly know our fate. It's a mystery. We can only live the best possible life because it goes pretty fast. Before you know it, your youth is gone and the next decade of your life is ever-present. What do you do when life passes you by? You start living your purpose immediately while you have the chance. The more purpose you discover in your life, the less depressed you become. If you get to the point where you experience success and depression finds its way back, reassess where the depression is coming from and release it from you. I have to tell myself this all the time because there is always a way out of the situation.

&

What is my purpose? This is a very important question because when you understand what you're here for, you'll begin creating light in the midst of darkness.

My purpose is to use my gift of writing to shed light for all the unheard voices; to create scholarship workshops to better inform students; to live purposeful with intention to experience greatness in my now, present moment; to pour out the gifts and talents God poured into me with a willing heart.

&

The levees of depression are broken in your life. All of the buildup you have been experiencing are being interrupted. The plans of the enemy will not work in your life, but you have to believe it. The chains have broken, so quit picking them back up. Do not allow confusion to infiltrate your mind. Be your own hero, and watch greatness elevate to your level. It all starts in the mind, so what are you putting in yours? Begin to cast those negative thoughts back to where they came from. Be intentional about your purpose, even if you're still discovering what that is. In all things, fight with both fists, declare power over your life and get back up when it all seems too overwhelming.

HOW ARE YOU DISCOVERING YOUR PURPOSE? WHAT'S YOURS?

_____

_____

_____

_____

_____

_____

_____

_____

_____

14

FINDING YOUR SAFE PLACE

"If you don't feel safe, you'll continue digging your grave.
Start shoveling greatness, and say to yourself:
these dry bones shall live."

I discovered at a very early age that I did not feel safe. I was twelve years old about to commit my first suicide attempt when it dawned on me that I was scared for my life. I believed that the only possible way to find safety was to end my life. I was so sure that I did not deserve to be here and I had no one telling me different. I cannot remember a time in my early childhood that I recall having a safe place to retreat to. I stated this before in a previous chapter, but I need to acknowledge that I joined a small church located in Los Angeles, California. It was there I found safety from the dangers of the streets and the heaviness of family. I was baptized on May 9th, 1999 at sixteen years old and began my journey to spiritual healing. During this time in my life, I found refuge in the arms of God, and although my struggles increased throughout the years, I continued fighting.

> *"I needed to find safety in God and myself so that I could become whole."*

In my opinion, when a person is experiencing high levels of depression, it is because they haven't found their safe place. I know this might sound strange, but although I found my safe place in the church as a teenager, it began to be uncomfortable. I was religiously going to church, marching in the choir, being active in the Youth and Young Adult Ministry, and attending service every time the doors were open. I was becoming so used to going to church that I overlooked the main things I needed in my life. I ignored the fact that I needed healing and restoration by constantly staying busy with church business. Don't misinterpret what you're reading. Church was still my safe place, but as I got older, I realized that I needed to find safety in God and myself so that I could become whole.

Finding safety for me first started with recognizing that I needed a relationship with the one I called my savior. I also needed to stop looking for it in people, and begin figuring out what I wanted in my life. I had an image in my mind of what I wanted to become, but it seemed unobtainable in my eyes at the time. *What did I want for my life?* At that point, the world became a blank canvas and I began stroking my dreams upon its surface, hoping to figure out who I was spiritually, mentally, emotionally, and physically.

◆———————◆

Spiritually: I was dead and open. I learned how to play church, but never learned how to nurture my spiritual being. I was like a mummy, walking around emotionless because I was guarded.

Mentally: I was depressed and suicidal. I had to go back in my life and pinpoint the root of my issues, which often left me vulnerable to any and everything.

Emotionally: I felt empty at times and did not know if I was worth the fight. I attempted to work out my emotions, but became overwhelmed and blocked people out of my life.

Physically: I felt unclean and damaged. I told myself that I was the dented can on the shelf that no one wanted.

This process took years to work through, and I am continuing the work to this day, *unashamed*. It does not matter how long it takes you, how many people you lose in your life, how many setbacks you have, or how empty you may feel at times. Remember, you are purging the dead weight out of your life, and sometimes it's going to hurt. What I can say is that it gets easier with time. If you are in this position right now, where you are trying to find the safe place within yourself, know that you are not alone. Take it one day at a time, and continue putting in the work. You must feel safe in all four of those areas I listed above in order to feel safe within your own skin. Start off by listing where you are now so that you can see what needs to be worked on. Take some time to figure out what you want to do in life, and don't worry about what others might say. The goal is to eliminate those areas in your life that are weighing you down. Keep track of your status by writing it down so that you can visually see where your *safe radar* is pointing. Start with this:

How do you feel?

Spiritually:

    _____

    _____

    _____

Mentally:

    _____

    _____

    _____

Emotionally:

- _____

- _____

- _____

Physically:

- _____

- _____

- _____

HAVE YOU FOUND YOUR SAFE PLACE?

15

SET GOALS

"Setting goals will help to boost your morale, and position you to being intentionally purposeful in your life."

*T*here was a time in my life that I would set certain goals for myself. I would have pages and pages of things I wanted to accomplish. A lot of people have these types of lists, which are commonly known as a *bucket list*. Since I have been training myself to think more positive, I choose not to call it a *bucket list* but instead, a *life list*. I say this because every day I am making a conscious choice to live. Making such a decision is rewarding in itself, but it's even greater when you are able to accomplish some things you desire. I have noticed that when most people write down their list, it often becomes a shadow of their past. For example, when you don't accomplish that goal, it becomes something you wanted to do, but never got around to doing it. This cycle needs to be broken.

> *"I had to fight and stop being intimidated by the mountain I am equipped to climb."*

Setting goals for yourself will help you when dealing with depression. I can only share my story because I am living proof of it. There was a time that I would write down my goals on my *life list*, but would never follow through. I started carrying self-doubt and my thoughts became so negative that I believed I wasn't designed for greatness. I believed that I did not have what it took to accomplish such goals and because of that I saw myself as a failure. The depression I experienced got heavier and I became an *inactive participate* in my life. You could say, I gave up. I crushed my dreams because I felt discouraged and I couldn't see a way out. At this point in my life, I tell myself all the time, "when the door is closed in your face, pick the lock." Don't allow your current situation to dictate what you are capable of.

After constant self-evaluation, I figured that I owed myself a chance to try. I had to fight and stop being intimidated by the mountain I am equipped to climb. I remember the first time I accomplished a goal I set for myself. I was twenty-two years old and had just moved to Sacramento, California. I had been working on my first book of poetry, "Mirror to my Soul", for quite some time. The more I focused on it, the more it became real in my life.

Here's a side note that just came to me: the more you focus on the negative it will become more real in your life. If you are wondering why your situation hasn't changed, maybe it's because you haven't changed your position.

I had decided that I was going to complete this goal no matter what, and soon enough I held the proof book in my hands. I couldn't believe it and was so excited that I shared with whoever I encountered. Completing that single goal boosted my morale and I became goal-oriented. I wanted to succeed! It became part of my desires for the future, and propelled me to keep going. Although I was experiencing moments of depression, setting and completing goals helped me to smile again. I reminded myself constantly that I deserved it, and I began accomplishing more goals that I set. Briefly, here are some major goals that I was able to accomplish:

- My first poetry book, *Mirror to my Soul* © 2005
- My second book, a memoir, *The Hush Language* © 2010
- Graduating with my AA degree in Liberal Arts, 2011
- Receiving my first scholarship, along with many more to follow, 2011
- Transferring to San Francisco State on Scholarship, 2011
- Studying Abroad at the University of East Anglia in Norwich, England, 2012
- Traveling throughout Europe, Italy, Paris and Amsterdam on scholarship, 2012-2013
- Graduating with my BA degree in English: Creative Writing, 2013
- Purchasing a brand-new car, 2013
- Moving into my own apartment after experiencing homelessness, 2014
- Publishing my third book, *The Scholarship Thief* © 2016
- Getting accepted into my MFA, Master's program, 2016

I am not trying to brag on my accomplishments per say, but I think that's the problem. I believe that you should brag about yourself and what you have accomplished. Don't worry about what anyone has to say concerning your life. Be present in who you are and set goals with the intention of seeing them to the end. The whole point of me sharing my above accomplishments is because depression had a good grip on me. It wasn't until I set goals and met them that I felt powerful in my skin, and no one could tell me different. Celebrate the small things in your life, and if depression is hovering over you, watch it begin to subside. You'll learn to be patient with your goals and not be too hard on yourself. This was one of the hardest lessons for me to learn, but I learned.

What are some goals you have set for yourself, and have accomplished them? Let's celebrate it.

  _____

  _____

  _____

  _____

  _____

  _____

  _____

  _____

  _____

What are some goals you wish to accomplish? For each one, list three things you could do to accomplish that goal.

🖋 ————————————————————————————————

————————————————————————————

————————————————————————————

————————————————————————————

🖋 ————————————————————————————————

————————————————————————————

————————————————————————————

————————————————————————————

🖋 ————————————————————————————————

————————————————————————————

————————————————————————————

————————————————————————————

16

FACING YOUR FEARS

"Being fearful causes you to miss out on opportunities, but facing your fears pushes you to create your own opportunity."

*I*n 2012, I journeyed back to my hometown of Los Angeles, California with a friend of mines. During this trip, I wanted to visit my nephews and my mom, as I do every year. When we arrived at my mom's apartment, I immediately felt the tension build up in chest. It was almost like something was sitting on me and for a few seconds I couldn't breathe. Although it seemed like a lifetime, I gathered my composure, got out of the car and made my way up the stairs to my mom's apartment. I was greeted with a warm hug by my nephews and that made me happy. As I entered the door, my sister who I do not have a relationship with, sat on the couch avoiding me. Sadly, we haven't been on speaking terms since I was a child, and never really had a sisterly bond. During this visit, I found the courage to say hello to her. There were a couple of things that I noticed about this moment. One, she didn't make any eye contact with me. Two, she couldn't find the courage in herself to respond. You may be thinking to yourself that this is odd behavior, and I would have to agree with you. Truth is, there are buried secrets hidden in plain sight in our *family*, and most of us are afraid to communicate. This is the case for all my siblings. We do not have a relationship with one another, and because it has been years, we have become strangers.

The fear I have always had growing up was not having a relationship with my siblings. It would bother me that I had three older sisters but could never go to any one of them about my problems. The older I got, and at this current point in my life right now, I have released that fear from within me. This may be hard for some of you to understand, but I chose not to have them in my life for various reasons. I do not want to go too in depth about this, but I will say that it was a hard decision for me, but a healthy one. I noticed that the more I kept the image of them not loving me growing up, the more I became sick and depressed. The more I thought about the abuse, the more I became angry. The more I held onto the lies, the more I became frustrated. I wanted the relationship with my sisters so bad growing up, but they never reached out to me and constantly rejected our relationship. When I allowed myself to feel certain ways, it affected the relationships I was trying to build with other people. I was harboring unhealthy characteristics because of the past hurts I experienced.

I went through a transition in my life because I was tired of carrying around the dead weight. I was becoming lifeless and knew I had to do something about it. This fear of desiring family and not having it was causing me to retreat backwards instead of forward. A couple of years ago, I released the poison out of my system and faced my fear on the throne of God by asking him to help me release whatever is making me sick. At certain times, I will revisit my journey to make sure that I am continuing on the right track.

What fears are you holding onto that are keeping you stagnant? If you're like me, and have dealt with a challenging childhood, then maybe you need to revisit that space in your mind and release it. I will not lie. It has been a difficult journey because there was so much I was holding onto. Regardless, I believe that I am worth fighting for and my destiny matters. If there are any fears you are standing up against, I challenge you to see yourself on the other side of it. Do not allow depression to keep you fearful of something that really has no control over your life. Be the hero of your own story, and show up for yourself. Eliminate your fear by praying against it. Say to yourself:

"This fear has no control over me. I see myself healthy, happy and whole. I believe that I am victorious over death, hell and the grave. I have a divine assignment and fear will not hold me back."

Repeat this until you have memorized it. When you feel like your back is up against the wall, and fear has got a grip on you, repeat it over your life. Honestly, I have gotten through some dark times in my life by speaking over myself. When you realize that your fear is powerless, you will become a better version of yourself. It amazes me when people say that they are proud of me, and encouraged by what I'm doing. They have no idea the secret battles I have come up against, and what I have just stepped out of. I have to constantly coach the inner me to continue pushing for greatness because if I didn't, I would be at home sitting on the bed with my head under the covers. I have to face my fears on a daily basis, and sometimes I really have to cry out to God for help. I hope you understand that you are not alone in this battle.

WHAT FEARS ARE YOU FACING?

17

SELF LOVE

"Loving yourself is greater than waiting on someone else to love you. When you're in this place of love, nothing else matters."

I believe that we should have another honest moment right now. Mainly because as we're coming to an end of this book, it is important that we talk about love. There were many times in my life that I felt loveless, unloved and unlovable. I will not mention any names, but I will say that there were some very important women in my life, who were like sisters, that I valued and made some mistakes with. Just like most of us, I had a lot of growing to do as a young woman trying to find herself, and I didn't always understand how to deal with certain situations. In those relationships, I allowed myself to get hurt because I was loving people over loving myself. At some point, I hit a crossroad and had to face the fact that our relationships were over. I always felt that as long as I had someone to love, I would be okay. I did not focus on loving who I was and because of it I drowned in my own self-pity.

> *"I have learned that self-love is about understanding who you are, so that you can treat yourself the way you should."*

One day I was browsing on YouTube and discovered this young lady, Abiola Abrams, a self-empowerment coach and entrepreneur, or spirit-preneur, as she says it. In her video, she discusses how important it is to display self-love daily. In the beginning, I would listen to her videos and say, "it's not that easy because I'm dealing with so much." The more she talked about self-love, the more I talked myself out of it. I continued watching her videos because I was intrigued that a beautiful brown *goddess (this is what she calls her subscribers)* was teaching women how to dig themselves up from a dark place. I realized that my negative talk was because I did not know how to love myself. I did not know where to begin, what to do, and how to do it. In the next video, she did something called EFT Tapping (Emotional Freedom Technique), which is also called energy tapping, for things such as anxiety healing, fear, obsessive worrying, rejection, getting unstuck, emotional freedom and so many more. I do not know much about EFT Tapping, but from what I witnessed, Abiola would center herself in a quiet place for meditation. As Abiola began, she would point to certain pressure points on her body to tap out anxiety and say, "even though I feel anxious, I choose to completely love, honor and cherish myself." Abiola would do this exercise while tapping her pressure points and speaking safety into her mind, body and soul. This is a wonderful way to start self-love. Another *ah-ha* moment. Whenever I felt low on energy, anxious or depressed I would trigger those pressure points and speak life back into my body. I guarantee that it works because of my personal experiences. If you wish to know more about EFT Tapping, please google and research information for your own needs. I am no expert, but I needed some emotional freedom on this self-love journey.

I have learned that self-love is about understanding who you are, so that you can treat yourself the way you should. For example, you wouldn't treat a queen any type of way because of who she is. This is the way you should look at yourself. I constantly remind myself that there is greatness inside of me and I am supposed to be here. Once I understood that my life is important, I began to treat myself better. I would speak well of myself, and like a magnet, others began to speak well of me. I would smile more and soon enough my peers would acknowledge the joy that's glowing from me. You have to find joy and rehearse it because if you can do it in private, it'll overflow in public. I began to treat myself the way I wanted others to treat me, and it showed. Here are some ways you can practice self-love:

- *Forgive yourself*: We have talked about forgiveness in an earlier chapter. It is important to release grudges so that you can move forward with your life. Remember, forgiveness is for you, not the other person.

- *Set boundaries*: Use your time wisely. You cannot do or be everything to everyone. Know when to say NO and be okay with your decision.

- *Live intentionally*: Wake up every morning with the intent to be courageous. Make your day count by speaking over yourself and having a positive attitude.

- *Become mindful*: Figure out what you want and take steps towards it. Keep your mind full of your ambitions and gravitate towards them.

- *Self-care*: Go and get a massage one day because you want to. Take a long walk and hike somewhere new. This challenged my thinking, and now I enjoy it.

- *Forget what other's think*: It does not matter what other people think of you. Live your life like there are no limits.

- *Surround yourself with loved ones*: Meet up with a friend for coffee and go window shopping. Honestly, I do this with a friend of mines frequently and we enjoy it. It is so therapeutic.

- *End toxic relationships*: Just like I mentioned above, you have to know when to release people out of your life. No matter how much I love them, I had to learn how to let go. Remember, everyone cannot go where you are going.

- *Celebrate small wins*: If you've accomplished a certain goal, stop by the ice cream shop and enjoy a couple scoops. I do this often as a reward and it makes me feel good.

- *Follow your passion*: If you want to be a writer, start writing – a singer, start singing – a dancer, start dancing. Whatever your passion is, do it while you can.

18

ACTION PLAN

*"Action plans allow you to redirect your energy
and prevent stagnation."*

*H*aving an action plan can really help when you experience bouts of depression. Throughout my life process, I have found that when I busy myself with what's important to me, it becomes easier to come out of darkness. The steps below can really help you, seriously. Do not doubt your process because something great may be at the end of it.

> Step One: *Determine Your Priorities*

Take a moment to list areas in your life that are most important to you. For example, some might say that family, financial security and health are important to them. After you've determined them, list three areas below, stating why they are important to you.

_____

_____

_____

_____

For each priority you listed above, figure out where you see yourself in the future in that area. I have done the first one for you as an example.

Priority	*1-2 years*	*5 years*	*End of Life*
Finances	*Debt paid off*	*Making more money*	*Financial freedom*

You may be asking yourself, *why do I have to list my priorities?* The reason, if you have not figured it out already, is because focusing on important areas in your life causes you to take action. When you take action over your life, you take control. When you have control, it is harder to allow depression, anxiety or stress to bring you down. You also should repeat this process throughout the years to make sure you are clear where you're going in life. You will start to see that you have low-tolerance for negativity, ignorance or pettiness because you are headed somewhere. Always ask yourself these questions: *What could I do to accomplish this goal? What is the reason I haven't succeeded? What can I do to succeed?* Never give up! Find a way to do what you are passionate about. This is just a simple action plan that has helped me to redirect my energy. There is power in writing things down and seeing it on paper.

Step Three: *Taking Action*

Once a month, or how frequent you desire, take one of your priorities and goals you listed above. Take actionable steps towards completing this goal and nurturing your priority. For example, you may choose finances as an action item during this month. I have done the first one for you.

Goal/Priority: Save $100 this month in my finances towards vacation. Taking a trip somewhere is a great way to escape from your surroundings and relax, all the while de-stressing your life.

Actionable Step 1:   Open a separate savings account and make your first deposit towards this goal. This will allow you to see your goal in progress during those difficult times.

Actionable Step 2:   Set up a direct transfer from your checking account to your new savings account each payday. If you get paid biweekly, you can put $50 each paycheck, or whatever amount you desire. When you are able to see your goal being completed, it creates momentum in your life.

On the next page, you have an opportunity to list your monthly goals and priorities for the month(s) you choose. You can choose to do this monthly, quarterly or every six months. I suggest that when you're first starting out, you do something towards your goal every month. For this exercise, there will be three months listed to get you started.

Month: _____

Goal/Priority (why?):

_____

_____

_____

Actionable Step 1 (how?):

_____

_____

_____

Actionable Step 2 (when?):

_____

_____

_____

Month:

Goal/Priority (why?):

_____

_____

_____

Actionable Step 1 (how?):

_____

_____

_____

Actionable Step 2 (when?):

_____

_____

_____

Month:_____

Goal/Priority (why?):

_____

_____

_____

Actionable Step 1 (how?):

_____

_____

_____

Actionable Step 2 (when?):

_____

_____

_____

For this note section, you can use it as a journaling device, diary of where you are and your improvement, or anything that comes to your mind worth jotting down. This section gives you plenty of room to be transparent enough to write it out of you.

NOTES

NOTES

NOTES

NOTES

NOTES

NOTES

NOTES

NOTES

NOTES

NOTES

I want to thank you for taking the time to hear part of my story, and for looking through my eyes for a moment. Understand that although depression can be tough, I am doing what it takes to continue living a successful life. Thank you for reading this book, and for supporting the cause of speaking out against depression, anxiety or any form of spirit that is not meant to be in your life.

Dear God,

I pray that the reader of this book finds healing and strength to go for their dreams, and continue to better their life's journey in discovering how great they are!

ABOUT THE AUTHOR

◆————————◆

A native of Los Angeles, California, *Toi Nichelle* began her career on a road that is rare amongst her peers. Having gone through challenges some would deem as traumatizing such as homelessness, abuse, neglect and suicidal attempts, she has cleared herself from the gates of low self-esteem to a balance of favor through faith. *"You can obtain the desires of your heart with a little hard work, sweat, patience and by not being afraid to fall when everyone is looking,"* she says when confronted with questions from those seeking advice.

It is not easy. As a matter of fact, you will come up against mountains which will make your dreams seem far beyond reach, but a leading example of perseverance is seen through *Toi Nichelle's* struggle. Within past years, *Toi Nichelle* has come from homelessness and mind-boggling low self-esteem. These situations gave her a reason to fight and run towards her destiny with no intent on giving up.

In 2007, she established Dream Loud Ink Publishing, which is in transition to publish material to heal our communities, and The Hush Language: A Young Girl's Breakthrough where she helps to encourage teens who struggle with abuse to move forward.

Toi Nichelle is a recipient of numerous scholarships some including, Kennedy King Scholarship, David Schirra Memorial Scholarship, Los Medanos Fund Scholarship and the Gilman Study Abroad Scholarship. She recently studied at the University of East Anglia in Norwich, England for an academic year, while touring through Europe to places like Paris, Italy and Amsterdam. *Toi Nichelle* has received her A.A. in Liberal Arts and Humanities from Los Medanos College (2011), and a B.A. in English: Creative Writing from San Francisco State University (2013).

Her professional goals include, developing as a business professional to be well equipped in all facets of life, and assisting with scholarship workshops to better inform students of various ages through her scholarship foundation, *The Scholarship Thief*; strengthening her social skills as an individual by connecting with like-minded people who are seeking to improve their personal standards of life; evolve as an inspirational speaker and writer to be the voice for so many young girls and boys who are silenced because of their childhood, ultimately helping them to find their way; and continuing to become a better person who fights with both fists.

Depression Wears Lipstick is her fourth book in print. *Toi Nichelle* currently resides in East Bay, California where she is surrounded by awesome friends and a powerful God.

RECOMMENDED BOOKS I'M READING

- The Bible

- "The Power of Now" – Eckhart Tolle

- "Purpose Driven Life" – Rick Warren

- "Abundance Now: Amplify Your Life and Achieve Prosperity

  Today" – Lisa Nichols

- "The Secret" – Rhonda Byrne

- "The Book of Esther" – Michelle McClain-Walters

HELPFUL RESOURCE LIST

> *Dealing with Depression*

- Suicide Hotline
  www.suicide.org
  (800) 273-8255

- The National Institute of Mental Health:
  www.nih.gov/health/depression

- National Alliance on Mental Illness:
  (800) 950-6264
  www.nami.org

- Anxiety and Depression Association of America:
  (240) 485-1001
  www.adaa.org

- National Institute of Mental Health:
  (866) 615-6464
  www.nimh.nih.gov

- American Psychiatric Association:
  (703) 907-7300
  www.psychiatry.org

Coping, Advocacy and Support

- American Foundation for Suicide Prevention:
  (800) 273-8255 / (800) 273-TALK
  www.afsp.org

- Depression and Bipolar Support Alliance:
  (800) 826-3632
  www.dbsalliance.org

- Families for Depression Awareness:
  (781) 890-0220
  www.familyaware.org

- To Write Love on Her Arms
  (800) 273-8255 / (800) 273-TALK
  www.twloha.com

Contact

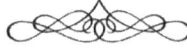

For bookings or to request Author Toi Nichelle for speaking engagements with youth and young adult groups, church groups and school assemblies please contact:

Mailing Address

Dream Loud Ink, Publishing
C/O Toi Nichelle
PO BOX 3411
Antioch, Ca 94509

Email

toi.nichelle@gmail.com
dreamloudinc@yahoo.com

PUBLISHER'S NOTE

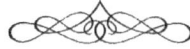

"Do you have a desire to be heard? Have a story you want to share? Don't know how to go about it?" Our motto: *"There are too many stories in the world that hold silence –too many voices go unheard. If we were all born quiet no one would speak. Trust your voice –tell the story."*

My name is Toi Nichelle, CEO and Founder of Dream Loud Ink –a company set to bring your imagination to paper. We are a publishing company geared towards creating a path for aspiring writers to be seen and heard throughout the literary community, while bridging the gap between voice and paper.

We are located in the Bay Area, but have an international reach seeking to connect with a massive audience in the urban inner-city communities and surrounding areas, to gain encouragement through our inspired writers. We are an inspired-based press-ready company helping self-publishers to produce uplifting material while being an encouragement in these hard-economic times.

Remember: *"A story seeks to follow in the footsteps of those who dare dream. One word on paper is a journey lived beyond the imagination."* We seek for that voice it seems no one is listening to.

We are currently taking consultations!

Email us at:

dreamloudinc@yahoo.com

www.ingramcontent.com/pod-product-compliance
Lightning Source LLC
Chambersburg PA
CBHW071127090426
42736CB00012B/2042